The Judo Advantage **Advance Praise**

"In this excellent volume by Steve Scott, he provides both the coach and the student with useful insights into just why and how the 'gentle way' functions as it does. I highly recommend that coaches and practitioners of judo carefully read this volume because it will enhance your coaching and judo practice."

—Jim Bregman
First US judo athlete to win Olympic and world medals
Bronze medalist, Tokyo Olympics, 1964
Bronze medalist, World Championships, 1965
US and Pan American Games judo champion

"In his new book on judo movement, Steve Scott has given a gift to all judoka. It is a tour de force regarding all the principles of judo. Unlike almost every other judo book, Steve does not try to tell you how he does—or thinks you should do—a particular throw, but rather gives an in-depth discussion of what is required to do any throw. Further, he shows how these principles often translate into newaza as well. It is a fitting adjunct text to the classic book *Canon of Judo*, by Kyuzo Mifune. I am looking forward to adding this wonderful text to my collection."

—Bruce Toups
Head coach, US team, World Judo Championships
Past director of development, United States Judo, Inc.
Coach of national and international judo champions

"Steve Scott has been there and done that. He knows what he is talking about. If you want to learn how and why judo works from someone who has been a successful coach for over forty years, read this book."

—AnnMaria DeMars, PhD
World and Pan American Games judo champion
US national judo champion
US national sambo champion

"Steve is not only my coach but my husband. I can tell you from personal experience that he has a deep understanding and appreciation of judo technical skill and how to coach it at all levels of competition, from teaching children to coaching at world-class tournaments."

—Becky Scott
World and Pan American Games sambo champion
US national judo champion
US national sambo champion

"This book explains how and why judo works and how to do it better. Whether you want to develop champions in any grappling sport or want to be a more effective coach teaching judo as physical education, I highly recommend that you read Steve's book."

—John Saylor
Three-time US national judo champion
Two-time Pan American medal winner
Head coach, US Olympic Training
Center judo team, 1983–1991
Director, Shingitai Jujitsu Association

"This book should be in the tool kit of any conscientious coach or aspiring judo coach as a comprehensible guide to understanding the fundamentals of judo and putting principles into practice. It would be near impossible to find all this information together in one place anywhere else. I know I will be putting it into my coaching practice as much as possible."

—Sophie Cox
Two-time judo Olympian for Great Britain
Four-time European medal winner
Seven-time British judo champion
World BJJ champion

"It is impossible to be involved in judo in the United States and not have heard of Steve Scott. Steve has been involved in the sport for decades, demonstrating over and over again that his knowledge and coaching ability are masterful. Not only does Steve continue to produce standout athletes, but he has achieved a much more challenging goal: training new generations of skilled coaches. Teaching people how to teach is a rare and valuable skill. Anyone interested in developing their technical arsenal and coaching ability must not overlook Steve Scott and all he has to offer. *The Judo Advantage* belongs on every judoka's bookshelf!"
—Stephen Koepfer
Head coach, New York Combat Sambo
Master of sport in combat sambo

"Steve Scott is my kind of coach. Every judoka can benefit from Steve's years of coaching experience and research. He uses a common-sense, grassroots approach to teaching."
—Bob Corwin
Head coach, Yorkville Judo Club US team coach,
World IJF Judo Championships (under 21)

"I know Mr. Steve Scott through my friend Gregg Humphreys. Steve invited me to do a sambo and judo clinic in Kansas City, USA. I was very impressed by Steve's technical knowledge and coaching record. I think he is a great coach. I think his books are good resource for any wrestler, sambo, judo, or jujitsu practitioner."
—Igor Kurinnoy
Three-time sambo world champion
Five-time Sambo World Cup champion

"It is an honor for me to recommend this new book by Steve Scott, one of the finest judo and jujitsu teachers I have ever met. His didactic methods are far beyond most of the teachings I have witnessed. Such a truly scientific approach to the instruction process is illustrated in his latest book, *The Judo Advantage*. I am sure all readers will deeply enjoy it an benefit from the knowledge packed in it."

—Ivica Zdravkovic, MD, PhD
President, Serbian Budo Council
Eighth dan, jujutsu; fifth dan, judo
International sport jujutsu champion

"When I explain to someone for the first time who Steve Scott is, I often describe him as a walking, talking judo encyclopedia and make that statement honestly and with respect. With this book, Steve has again proven my description to be an accurate one. It is obvious that he has a deep and far-reaching pool of judo knowledge. It is this deep understanding that allows him to easily and succinctly break down such a complex subject as judo. I teach judo every day as the head coach of a large judo club and value books such as this one that provide realistic and practical information. This book is an excellent addition to the resource library of any student or teacher of any of the grappling arts, and I highly recommend it."

—James Wall
Owner, Wall to Wall Martial Arts, Denham Springs, Louisiana

"I have known Steve Scott for over thirty years. In that time I've come to know him as a superb judo, sambo, and jiu-jitsu coach. He has trained multiple world, Pan American, and national champions in each discipline. In his latest book, *The Judo Advantage*, he explains the concepts of the grappling sports and why they work. This book will give you an understanding of principles and methods of training and why we do them. Whether you're a coach, competitor, or just a fan of the grappling sports, this book will give you a greater understanding and appreciation of them."

—Gregg Humphreys
Judo, sambo, and Shingitai coach
Dynamo Combat Club

THE JUDO ADVANTAGE

Also by Steve Scott

Sambo Encyclopedia

Triangle Chokes: Triangle and Leg Chokes for Combat Sports

Vital Jujitsu (with John Saylor)

Juji Gatame Encyclopedia

Winning on the Mat

Conditioning for Combat Sports (with John Saylor)

Tap Out Textbook

Groundfighting Pins and Breakdowns

Drills for Grapplers

Throws and Takedowns

Grappler's Book of Strangles and Chokes

Vital Leglocks

Championship Sambo: Submission Holds and Groundfighting

Championship Sambo (DVD)

Armlock Encyclopedia

Juji Gatame Complete (with Bill West)

Coaching on the Mat

THE
JUDO
ADVANTAGE

STEVE SCOTT

YMAA Publication Center
Wolfeboro, New Hampshire

YMAA Publication Center, Inc.
PO Box 480
Wolfeboro, New Hampshire, 03894
United States of America
1-800-669-8892 • info@ymaa.com • www.ymaa.com
ISBN: 9781594396281 (print) • ISBN: 9781594396298 (ebook)
Copyright © 2019 by Steve Scott
All rights reserved including the right of reproduction in whole or in part in any form.
Managing editor: T. G. LaFredo
Editor: Doran Hunter
Cover design: Axie Breen
This book typeset in Adobe Garamond and Frutiger
Typesetting by Westchester Publishing Services

Illustrations courtesy of the author, unless otherwise noted.

POD0719

Publisher's Cataloging in Publication

Names: Scott, Steve, 1952– author.
Title: The judo advantage : controlling movement with modern kinesiology / by Steve Scott.
Description: Wolfeboro, NH USA : YMAA Publication Center, Inc., [2019] | Includes bibliographical references.
Identifiers: ISBN: 9781594396281 (print) | 9781594396298 (ebook) | LCCN: 2018964054
Subjects: LCSH: Judo—Training. | Judo—Physiological aspects. | Martial arts—Physiological aspects. | Wrestling—Physiological aspects. | Kinesiology. | Biomechanics. | Human mechanics. | Human locomotion. | Hand-to-hand fighting—Training. | Martial arts—Training. | Wrestling—Training. | BISAC: SPORTS & RECREATION / Martial Arts & Self-Defense. | SPORTS & RECREATION / Training. | SPORTS & RECREATION / Wrestling.
Classification: LCC: GV1114.33.T72 | DDC: 796.815/3—dc23

CONTENTS

INTRODUCTION

Judo is based on sound biomechanical principles. The more efficiently a person applies these principles, the more effectively that person will do judo. To do judo well, a person must know not only how to control his own body but also his opponent's. This book examines how the human body moves and why judo works in controlling how it moves.

We will examine and analyze this from both a contemporary biomechanical point of view and from a more "traditional" point of view, with the goal of showing how both these ways of describing what judo is are compatible and make a lot of sense. The Japanese phrases, terms, and names you'll encounter—in use since judo's inception and familiar to all judo practitioners—explain much of what judo is and does. You just have to appreciate them and use them to explore the fullness and complexity of the art. For the most part, terms such as kuzushi, tsurikomi, and many others—terms we often use without giving them much thought—are based on sound biomechanical principles. Words do indeed have meaning and purpose and, for the most part, the Japanese names in judo translate into functional application. Typical examples are kuzushi, tsukuri, and kake. These well-known terms describe both a physical action and the theoretical concept behind that physical action. Kuzushi translates to "breaking down" and describes the action of breaking down an opponent's balance and posture. Tsukuri translates to "building or erecting" something and describes the attacker's action of building or forming his technique. Kake translates to "suspend, hoist, or raise" and describes how the attacker raises or suspends his opponent up off the mat in the actual execution of the attack. The meanings of the terms neatly describes the action involved.

Controlling how an opponent moves is vital to success in judo, as well as in any other combat sport. Judo is movement. A judo practitioner must be able to control how his own body moves but has the added burden of controlling how his opponent moves as well. Making your opponent move the way you want him to and controlling as much of what goes on in a judo match determine who wins and who loses. Make no mistake about it: judo is one of the toughest sports ever invented. Judo is also an effective method of developing fitness and health, useful for self-defense, and ideal for developing a sound character. But when it comes down to it, if you want to be good at judo, you have to know how to move an opponent and move him with a high ratio of success.

Controlling the movement of a partner in practice is different than controlling the body movement of an uncooperative and resisting opponent in a judo match. For a technical skill to be effective in a competitive situation, there has to be a reliable foundation for it. This foundation is the physical education aspect of judo. The biomechanical principles that are the foundation of how and why judo works in a sporting context are the same principles that govern judo as a method of study in physical education.

Throughout my coaching career, I've used the phrase "control judo" to describe how to effectively teach the functional movements necessary for success in judo. The basic idea is for the athlete (and the coach who prepares that athlete) to control as much of the action in a match as possible. In any conflict with another human being, you must control every aspect of that conflict, and you must leave nothing to chance. Whether in competition or self-defense, controlling an opponent is the ultimate goal.

While this book may appear to emphasize judo's competitive aspect, the fact remains that judo is first and foremost a method of physical education. A major part of physical education is the teaching of good sportsmanship. Good sportsmanship is basically good ethics applied to a sport. These good ethics taught on the mat are what develop good character and a decent human being. Judo's founder, Professor Jigoro Kano, placed primary emphasis on judo as physical education and secondary emphasis on judo as a sport.

That said, millions of people all over the world practice judo as a competitive sport. Judo's expansion from Japan to the rest of the world has been mostly due to people pursuing judo as the exciting sport that it is. From a technical point of view, judo's development has come largely from the coaches and athletes who compete in it. All of these people have pushed the envelope in search of improved technical skills to get the edge on opponents. Judo tests and pushes the boundaries of human movement. What allow those boundaries to be pushed are the sound biomechanical principles rooted in the physical education aspect of judo. Without its foundation in physical education, judo as a sport would not be the technically compelling activity it is today.

Judo was my first exposure to the world of martial arts. I was twelve. But along the way I developed keen interests in both jujitsu and sambo and am a firm believer in the concept of cross-training. Judo and similar combat sports are complex activities based on sound biomechanical principles and each art provides its own perspective that is worth exploring. But historically, judo is the root discipline of most of today's combat grappling sports, and because of this, I will use judo as the primary sport when I explain the biomechanics of a technical skill or movement.

The principles of judo initially developed by Professor Jigoro Kano have stood the test of time because everything he did was based on sound biomechanical principles. Throughout this book you will see familiar judo terminology alongside terms used in kinesiology and biomechanics. This book is not an attempt to reinvent the wheel or even to make it rounder. Rather, this book simply attempts to explain why the wheel works. As mentioned, much of the Japanese terminology in judo most students tend to take for granted is based on fundamentally sound concepts. These concepts are considered "old school" but have stood the test of time because they continue to explain why and how the human body works most efficiently in the context of judo. Along the same lines, one of the most brilliant things Jigoro Kano did was to give a descriptive name to each of the different actions in judo. An example is shintai. Shintai is the term used to describe movement, most usually in a linear pattern. From that, we have the different footwork or movement patterns of ayumi ashi, or normal walking; tsugi ashi, or shuffling footwork; and taisabaki, or body movement in a circular pattern. Each of these movement patterns are part of the overall concept of shintai.

From my research, prior to Jigoro Kano and Kodokan judo, no hand-to-hand fighting art (such as the different feudal Japanese jujutsu schools) had specific names for specific movements based on their function. Professor Kano largely brought this method of describing things to the names he gave to the different throws, pins, strangles, and armlocks in Kodokan judo. For the most part, the name of a technique provides a description as to how that technique should optimally work. This pragmatic, simple, and logical concept of naming things has ensured that the biomechanical principles of Kano's judo have stood the test of time with continued success. The Japanese language is considered to be the common language used to describe the techniques, theory, and concepts of judo much in the same way Latin is used in science and law. This has helped tremendously in the promulgation, teaching, and explaining of judo. If the Japanese terminology were no longer used, much of the analytical understanding and appreciation of judo would be lost. It is a good idea for any serious student of judo (or similar martial art) to learn and understand the Japanese names and phrases to better appreciate the underlying concept of a particular movement or technique. A person doesn't have to speak or read Japanese fluently, but it does take an accurate understanding of the terms to better understand what a particular name or phrase really means. As noted, in most cases Professor Kano named things based on their function. One of this book's main purposes is to explain what these names mean and how the principles they describe actually work.

Judo is kinesiology in action. Kinesiology is the study of the human body's movement, and that describes judo very well. Knowing how to control an opponent's body and then actually doing it defines success in judo. Movement and the control of movement are what keep judo practitioners up at night, and I am no different. I certainly am not an academic, but I do possess a fair amount of education, practical training, and experience in how to make a human body work and how to do so optimally under the stress of training and competition. It is safe to say that all books stand on the work of those who have come before them. This book too is based on the work of many authors, coaches, and technicians along with my own analysis. My purpose is to succinctly explain in one volume how and why judo works. But I highly recommended that you go out and study as many different sources as possible, especially the references listed in this book. I am writing from the perspective of a coach who has had a good amount of experience coaching at both the club level as well as at the international level, and who has been fortunate enough to have travelled to many places and met many people in my pursuit of judo, sambo, jujitsu, and submission grappling. The contents of this book are merely my sincere but limited contribution to the existing body of knowledge.

STEVE SCOTT

A FEW WORDS ABOUT USING THIS BOOK

In the chapters ahead, key words and phrases are in bold lettering. In some instances, these may be repeated based on the context of what is being discussed. Terminology conventionally used in judo will be interspersed with terminology definitively used in the study of human movement in order to provide more clarity. Additionally, the photos in this book show athletes and coaches in both judo and sambo uniforms, and others show athletes in "no gi" situations. Please do not be surprised if what looks like a judo technique is performed by people who are wearing sambo uniforms or vice versa. A good move is a good move, no matter what sport it's done in or what type of clothing people are wearing.

FOREWORD BY JIM BREGMAN

The genius of Dr. Kano's creation, judo, is fully unlocked and thoroughly analyzed in this exploration and explanation of controlling movement by Steve Scott. Seiryoku zenyo, which can be best translated as "the best use of energy or maximum efficiency with a minimum of effort" is one of Dr. Kano's guiding principles. The other is jita kyoei, which is translated as "mutual welfare and benefit." The word judo is often translated as the "gentle way."

As a form of physical education and sport, judo provides an excellent vehicle for imparting in its practitioners a practical code of conduct and deportment that is crystallized in the phrase "mutual welfare and benefit." As judo's practitioners become more and more developed and trained in this more modern form of a martial art, they begin to have greater insight into the full meaning of "maximum efficiency with a minimum of effort." In this excellent volume, Steve Scott provides both the coach and the student with useful insights into just why and how the gentle way functions as it does.

At the age of fifteen, I was awarded my shodan rank and competed in the regional tournament held by Shufu Judo Yudanshakai. I won my division and became the overall tournament champion by throwing the heavyweight champion for an ippon with uchi mata. Despite my larger and heavier opponent, the throw was effortless due to body mechanics and, philosophically, mushin or "mindlessness." Mushin happens when the thrower is not consciously thinking and is "mindless" as the activity is occurring. This mindlessness is an automatic reflex developed by years of repetitive practice and diligence. These principles are included in this book.

The axiom that a much smaller man can defeat a bigger opponent is explained by body dynamics and movement control. Although I was successful as a fifteen-year-old defeating a much stronger and heavier opponent, I learned very quickly watching Anton Geesink (world and Olympic champion) train at the Kodokan and doing randori with him that the real principle at work in this case was "the bigger they are, the harder they throw you." You will learn why this is true as you enjoy Steve's insightful comments about how judo really functions.

I highly recommend that coaches and practitioners of judo read this volume because it will enhance and amplify your coaching and judo practice.

JIM BREGMAN
US and Pan American Games judo champion
First US judo athlete to win world and Olympic medals
Tenth dan

FOREWORD BY BRUCE TOUPS

In his new book on judo movement, Steve Scott has given a gift to all judoka. It is a tour de force regarding all the principles of judo. Unlike almost every other judo book, Steve does not try to tell you how he does, or thinks you should do, a particular throw, but rather discusses in depth what is required to do *any* throw. It is a fitting adjunct to Kyuzo Mifune's classic book *Canon of Judo*. Further, Steve shows how these principles often translate into newaza (ground grappling) as well.

This book should be in everyone's library. Why? First, it is a summary of everything a good judo teacher or coach should know as well as a reference text to help all of us remember the things we know but have forgotten to emphasize to our students in our lesson plans, because we are concentrating on a particular technique rather than its principles.

I am looking forward to adding this wonderful text to my collection. However, unlike most of the books I have, this one will be nearby for reference.

BRUCE TOUPS
US World Judo Team coach
Past director of development for US Judo
Seventh dan

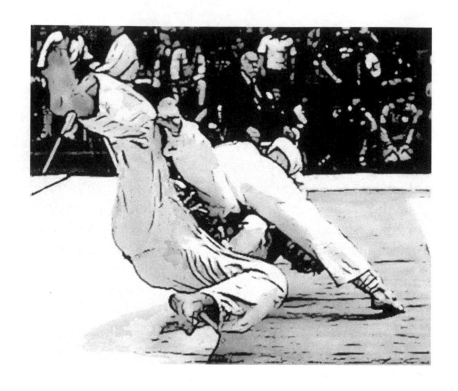

"The key to effective judo is movement."

—James Bregman

CHAPTER 1

Judo as Kinesiology

Judo as Kinesiology—The Study of Human Movement within the Context of Judo

The two primary aspects of controlling an opponent and his movement are tactical and, most importantly, physical. Tactical applications need a sound biomechanical basis.

Contest rules are written with the biomechanical movements of judo in mind, while tactical considerations are based on whatever the current contest rules permit and do not permit. In a sporting context, coaches teach according to how the rules are written. This book's focus is on the physical movements of judo and the biomechanical principles of how to control movement and why these principles work. The contest rules of

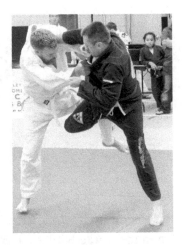

judo have changed considerably over the years, but what doesn't change is the fact that good judo is good judo, no matter what the rules are. A skillful technique that worked in 1964 still works today, and that's because, while the rules may change, the way the human body works doesn't change.

Impose Your Will on Your Opponent

There is a method to our madness. Judo is based on sound scientific methodology. Our task as coaches and serious students is to learn, understand, and apply as much of this methodology as possible and to teach it to our students in a way they will be able to understand and apply with a high rate of success. The reason controlling movement is fundamentally important is simple: in any form of sport combat, the primary goal is to impose your will on your opponent—in other words, to make your opponent fight your kind of fight. The only way to do this is to control your opponent and, in order to control your opponent, you must control how he moves.

The Primary Physical Purpose of Judo Is to Control Movement

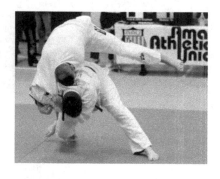 In judo, or any combat sport for that matter, the opponent has the same goal as you. He wants to control you just as much as you want to control him. Like you, he's fit, motivated, and skilled and has every intention of doing to you what you want to do to him. Success in judo depends on the optimal application of technical skill and the biomechanical forces underlying that skill. The goal is to throw, pin, choke, or

armlock a resisting and motivated opponent. Fundamentally, the primary purpose of judo, sambo, and similar sports is to control movement. The better an athlete controls his movement and the movement of his opponent, the better the result will be for him. Good skill and all the factors that comprise it are based on controlling movement. With that in mind, this book describes some of the fundamental principles behind controlling movement coaches can use to prepare students and athletes for success in judo.

Judo Is the Practical Application of Kinesiology

Judo, in a very real sense, is the study of human movement, and this is a useful definition of kinesiology. This book is not meant to be a textbook on either kinesiology or biomechanics. However, since judo is based on sound biomechanical principles, the contents of this book will combine modern concepts of kinesiology and dynamics with many of Kodokan judo's time-honored technical theories and practices to confirm that judo does indeed provide a unique and functional approach to physical education and sport. So then, let's look at some basic definitions necessary to appreciating how to better control movement in judo.

Kinesiology: A basic definition of kinesiology is that it is the study of movement as well as the study and understanding of mechanics and anatomy relative to the movement of the human body. The word is Greek in origin and literally means "movement study." One application of kinesiology that is relevant to our analysis is biomechanics.

Biomechanics: One basic definition relevant to our analysis and use of biomechanics is that it is the study of force and the effect force has on the human body in sport as well as in exercise. It is a subset of **mechanics**, which is the study of the effects of forces acting on objects. Specifically, our interest in how this relates to judo is in the study of **rigid body mechanics**, which explains the gross movements of a human body. This is further divided into the concept of **statics**, which is the mechanics of a body at rest and constant velocity, and **dynamics**, which is the concept of a body or object in accelerated motion. As coaches and serious students of judo, a college-level study of biomechanics or kinesiology is not necessary, but it is important for us to comprehend the basic concepts of why and how judo works and to know that it is firmly rooted in science. Our primary focus in doing judo is how to efficiently and practically put to use the conceptual theories of dynamics and, as coaches, to understand dynamics. These are the core concepts of why and how judo works as efficiently as it does.

To better understand biomechanics, a brief look at Sir Isaac Newton's laws is helpful. Always keep in mind that judo is based on the laws of gravity. A person doesn't have to memorize these laws, but it's a good idea to understand them and know how they apply to judo. Newton formulated three laws of motion and the law of gravitation, which form the basis of modern mechanics—and, more important to our discussion, the basis of biomechanics. Newton's Laws tell us about force, gravity, how an object reacts when force is applied to it, and the source of external force. Newton's Laws of Motion basically are:

1. Every object stays at rest or moves in the same direction unless that object is made to change by an outside force. This law describes inertia.

2. Changes in momentum of an object (for us, a human body) are the direct result of the force applied to the object. The change in momentum will go in the same direction as the force that has been applied. Any change in a body's motion depends on the mass of that body. It is force that causes a change in the speed and direction of a human body.

3. For every action, there is an opposite and equal reaction.

Also, Newton's Law of Gravitation basically states that two bodies or objects are attracted to each other with a force directly proportional to their masses and inversely proportional to the square of the distance between them. In other words, the more massive the bodies, the more gravitational force between them, and the farther away they are, the less gravitational force between them.

Kodokan judo provides a practical biomechanical framework for the study and application of kinesiology. Kinesiology, the study of movement, explains why judo works. As stated previously, judo works because it is based on sound biomechanical principles. This book simply explains these principles and how they can be efficiently used in the teaching, learning, practice, and application of judo.

A coach has the responsibility to clearly teach these principles to his athletes and students so they become habitual. Teaching fundamentals based on sound biomechanical principles is not a task to be taken lightly. A coach at any level has a serious responsibility, but the role of the club coach is especially vital. It's the club coach who first introduces a beginning student to the movements of judo. If the club coach teaches these fundamental movements poorly, the beginning student has little chance of ever attaining mastery.

Without good fundamentals, no one can proceed to more advanced skills. Few people, if any, have the ability to leapfrog immediately to advanced applications of body movement and technical skill without having a solid grasp of the basic movements of judo. Learning the many complex biomechanical skills that comprise judo takes place gradually and sequentially.

Reaction Time: This is the amount of time it takes for a body to respond to a stimulus. **Movement Time:** This is related and is the time it takes for a body to carry out a movement. The faster the reaction time, the faster the movement time will be. In other words, the faster the nervous system perceives something happening, the faster it will react by performing a movement. For a judo technique to be efficiently applied, the person doing it must have a heightened reaction time. The body moves because its muscles contract to manipulate the bones they are attached to at the joints. The central nervous system sends messages to the brain, then to the spinal cord, and then to the motor nerves that run through the muscles and cause the muscles of the body to contract. The stimulus is accepted at the joint nerve center and is changed into messages. The time it takes for these messages to be carried to the motor nerves is what is known as reaction time. If the same stimulus is given repeatedly, the reaction time lessens or quickens. This means that the more a body is exposed to something, the quicker it responds to it. This is how repetition training works. If the athlete repeats a movement over and over, the nervous system will cause the body to react faster.

Instinctive and Automatic Response: The body's natural response to any stimulus is called an instinctive response. Through training, a human body can be habituated to react to a stimulus in a specific way as an automatic response. Sometimes an instinctive response is the right one, but in just as many cases (especially in judo) it's not. An instinctive response is a natural or unconditioned reflexive action and an automatic response is a learned or conditioned reflexive action. Athletes can learn reflexes that are either optimal or suboptimal, correct or incorrect. The goal is to train oneself to react optimally and automatically in as many situations as possible. This allows the athlete to reflexively use the best judgment when performing the technique. In the same way, learning to ride a bicycle is difficult at first but soon becomes second nature. Though we must ride it regularly to keep up our skill, we don't need to learn to ride it all over again every time. In other words, a person learns to ride a bicycle by being taught the right way to ride it and then by maintaining that skill through practice. There is more on this a bit later in an examination of repetition.

Decreased Reaction Time: Reaction time is decreased or slowed in several situations. One of the most common situations is when an athlete is physically fatigued. A tired athlete will not react as quickly to an opponent's attack or take advantage of an opening. Optimal technical skill is based on optimal physical fitness. Another instance where reaction time decreases is when an athlete is emotionally upset or under stress that is too much for him to handle. This is why the coach should place more stress on his athletes in training than they will encounter in an actual tournament. Another instance when reaction time is less than optimal is when an athlete has his attention focused on the wrong thing at the wrong time. This is how a feint works in a renraku waza (combination technique). An attacker will feint a movement to distract the defender. When the defender focuses on that distraction, the attacker launches his major attack. When multiple stimuli are applied, the athlete's reaction decreases. In other words, an athlete who attacks a physically fatigued opponent with a combination attack will have better success than if he attacks a physically fit opponent with the same combination attack. Another situation when response or reaction time is decreased is when the practitioner is not skilled or is untrained in judo. This is why novices are generally not competitive with more advanced athletes in any sport, not just judo. Beginners simply don't know how or when to react. In some cases, if a novice has naturally good reflexes and strength, he may be competitive with a more skilled (but possibly poorly conditioned) opponent.

Mastery of Skill: In the martial arts, when people mention the word "master," the image that comes to mind might be an old man with a wispy white beard who can defeat all opponents and hands out sage advice. Out of humility, a lot of people don't use the word "master" because it's believed that "mastering" something is an impossible task; mastery for them means perfection. And, in one sense of the word, that is accurate. However, to master a skill is to have command over all of the parts, as well as of the whole, of that skill. Mastery is understanding why and how something works and being able to apply it. Breaking down the steps or parts of any skill requires a logical and progressive method of instruction and learning. As a student learns the basic physical application of a technique and progresses in his learning, he begins to better understand and appreciate the principles that make a specific technique work and work most efficiently. Once the fundamental biomechanical framework of a technique is learned and the student gains confidence in his basic application of it, he must adapt it so it works best for him. But it has to be stressed that the student must first be able to physically perform and apply the technique with proper biomechanics before he can go on to adapt it to fit his body type and personalize it to make it most functional for him. Once this is achieved, it takes thousands of repetitions of the movement to master it.

Repetition: A repetition is something done more than once. In the context of the mastery of a skill, it is a movement repeated in the most efficient way for the person doing it under the conditions he must do it in. Conversely, an athlete can do thousands of repetitions of a particular throw, but if he does them in a way that is technically incorrect or not biomechanically efficient, he will never be able to effectively use that throw. Repeating something—anything—thousands of times creates permanence. In learning skills, the key is to create permanence through the most efficient and effective application of the skill one wants to master.

Style: What is known as style is the personal touch an athlete gives to a technique or movement pattern. Style is functional or applied skill that makes a technique work most efficiently for the person doing it. Style can only be achieved after a student has a thorough understanding of, and ability to perform, the basics.

Every human body is different and it takes many hours of hard, concerted effort to personalize a technique so it works best for the person doing it. As Miles Davis said, "You have to play a long time to be able to play like yourself."

Optimal: You will see this word used frequently in this book (we've seen it a few times already). Optimal is defined as "the most favorable point, degree, or amount of something for obtaining a given result in a situation." For our purposes, when an athlete performs a technique with optimal skill, he is doing it in the most efficient manner that works best for him in the situation for which it is intended. This efficient application becomes an effective application, often with a high ratio of success. The application of the technique is functionally efficient and effective relative to the circumstances in which it is used.

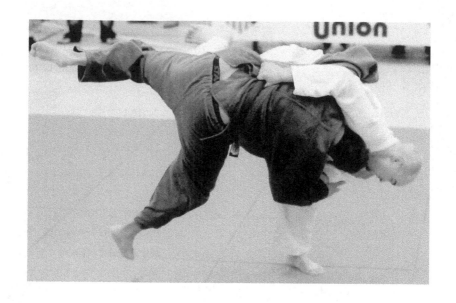

"Make the technique work for you."

—Maurice Allan, MBE

CHAPTER 2

Judo Relies on Both Power and Skill

Judo Techniques Rely on Both Power and Skill

Some people mistakenly believe that power is bad in judo—that good technique does not require power. In fact, the opposite is true.

Power is necessary for technical skill. Anything that requires energy to perform, including the application of a judo technique, requires power. There must be some source of energy that makes things happen, and power is that source of energy. Power is the application of physical strength (force) combined with speed and the controlled direction of movement (velocity). So let's delve into how power and skill combine to produce a technically sound movement.

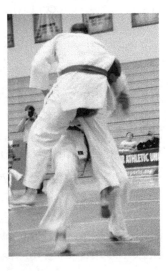

Power: A basic definition of power is the amount of mechanical effort required to produce a desired effect. It's force multiplied by how fast it is applied and in the direction you apply it. A fast, direct effort produces more force than a slow, indirect effort. For our purposes, power is a focused combination of speed and strength. In a strict sense, it is velocity (speed and direction) combined with functional strength and performed with ballistic effect.

This combination of applying muscular force with velocity creates **momentum**. Momentum is the power used to throw an opponent. To some judo practitioners, the word "power" implies brute strength, but this is not what power is. The bottom line is that a person must have sufficient functional strength and speed in order to perform any judo technique, especially a highly skilled and complex movement such as a throwing technique.

Force: Biomechanically, force equals mass times acceleration. This is a push, pull, or other movement the attacker uses to change the state of motion of the defender's body. This is what is known as **action force.**

In other words, the action of the attacker driving off one or both feet when performing a throwing technique creates force. When that force is directed with speed and in a specific direction, it creates momentum. This action creates power, and power is necessary for optimal application of every technical skill in judo. There is more about force in the section relating to torque later in this book.

The Concept of "Ju": A core concept in judo that deserves analysis is *ju*. The popular translation of ju is "soft," and while partly accurate, this translation gives an incomplete (and often downright inaccurate) picture of what ju is. The idea that a soft, weak, or poorly conditioned person will be able to throw a larger opponent who is resisting, fit, and motivated is simply not based in reality. It takes the work of Jigoro Kano out of context and vastly oversimplifies it. This oversimplification of Kano's conception of the "softness" of judo has been used for years to attract new students.

The word ju with the corresponding kanji ideograph translates to "gentle, mild, soft, flexible, yielding, or pliant" (the same ideograph and meaning is used for yawara, a method of self-defense native to Japan). In fact, Kano even referred to the word "gentle" as the underlying principle of his invention numerous times. What Professor Kano intended by using the term ju is clear. Judo is not based on brute strength but rather on rational scientific principles for the application of power and controlling balance (and, as a result, controlling movement) and the most efficient use of both physical and mental abilities. Kano was a pragmatist and stressed the most efficient use of energy. He created the maxim **seiryoku zen'yo**, which means "the best use of energy" and this became the foundation for the principle of ju.

When Professor Kano began his studies in jujutsu, he was not athletically gifted. He was rather small and weak physically, and like a lot of other young men, wanted to learn how to defend himself. During his study of jujutsu, he became interested in understanding why the various throws and holds worked against larger and stronger opponents. To his pragmatic way of thinking, there had to be a biomechanical reason that throwing techniques worked. Eventually, he developed the concept of kuzushi as the reason, with the underlying principle of ju as kuzushi's foundation. Kuzushi is the reason ju works. Along with optimal application of tsukuri and kake, kuzushi provides the structure and methodology for teaching and learning technical skill in throwing (as well as in newaza, since these principles apply to groundfighting too).

Professor Kano's belief that "softness can overcome hardness" provides the rational biomechanical and tactical reason for why judo works. It is the best use of energy. In Chinese military strategy, "softness" is the ability to be adaptable and flexible and to use every means possible to defeat the enemy. "Hardness" refers to an inability to be adaptable—to be rigid both physically and tactically.

Judo Isn't Gentle

In reality, judo isn't "gentle" in the popular sense of that word. Judo is rough and tumble—one of the most demanding of all sports. Anyone who has seriously studied and practiced judo for any significant amount of time can attest to this.

The most efficient use of power is a necessary component in the application of technical skill in judo. This efficient use of power translates into results. "Ju" is the most efficient use of physical and mental energy because it is adaptable, flexible, and pragmatic. This is why judo has stood the test of time. It is the responsibility of coaches to train their athletes properly so they can make the most effective use of power when they need it. Ju is the efficient application of power (or, as Professor Kano explained, it is "directed energy"). It is my opinion that this is what Professor Kano meant by "ju." "Gentle" and "soft" do not do justice to the concept of ju.

Professor Kano taught that for the purposes of throwing an opponent, sometimes the more direct principle of leverage is more important than giving way. He said that judo's true essence is making the most efficient use of mental and physical energy. The use Professor Kano made of the concepts of ju and kuzushi reflect his innovative brilliance. Ju was, and remains, the central theme of his invention, Kodokan judo, in 1882. He believed in the concept so much that he named his invention judo, the "way or philosophy of ju."

Ju Relies on a Sound and Fit Body

For the principles of ju and kuzushi to be effective, the person applying them must be physically fit. Of two contestants with the same skill level, the one who is better conditioned will tend to win. Conversely, the closer two contestants are in fitness and conditioning, the one who is more skillful will probably win. This shows how dependent fitness and skill are on each other and, more specifically, how important fitness is in the application of kuzushi, which produces effective skill. Another critical factor in controlling movement and the concept of ju is how well the athlete maximizes his power and transfers it efficiently to his technical skill. In actuality, this is exactly what Professor Kano was getting at with his description of ju. For example, a trained and fit 135-pound athlete will not be as physically strong or powerful as a trained and fit 235-pound athlete if for no other reason than that the smaller athlete cannot generate enough force based on his smaller physical size. However, if the smaller athlete maximally and efficiently transfers his power to his technical ability and does so better than his larger opponent, he will be better able to perform his technical skills and possibly beat his larger opponent. In other words, the smaller athlete, as Teddy Roosevelt said, "does the best he can with what he has and where he's at." This is sage advice for judoka. It is critical that athletes mold or adapt the technique to their personal requirements so they can maximize their power and make as skillful an application of the technique as possible.

Skill: Skill is how a technique is applied. For our purposes, skill refers to the practical and most efficient application of technique. A skillful technique is the effective application of that technique, and for a technique to be effective, it must be 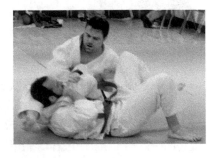 molded to work for the athlete with the highest rate of success possible. Skill is the optimal application of a technique specifically suited to the person performing it. When someone comments favorably about a judoka, he may say "he has good technique." This really means that the judoka is skilled at performing techniques.

Conversely, a technique can be performed with poor skill. This occurs when the athlete does not have an adequate grasp of the basic structure or purpose of the technique or how to apply it in the most efficient way possible.

Power provides the physical base and skill provides the technical base of every movement in judo, sambo, or any grappling sport. If an athlete has power but minimal skill, or if an athlete has skill but minimal power, he or she will not be successful. Power and skill are interdependent; neither is more important than the other. For an athlete to be successful in judo, both power and skill are necessary.

Skill doesn't happen in a vacuum and doesn't just magically appear. Skill is the practical, optimal, and functional application of technique under realistic, stressful, competitive circumstances (or in self-defense). The athlete who most efficiently and effectively combines power and technical skill will prevail.

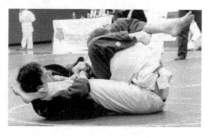
When something is seen as "skillful," it's because the movement being performed is done with functional efficiency. In other words, if a technique is done with skill, it's done in the most efficient manner possible to achieve the goal at hand or get the job done. This is how a technique, which is a distinct movement pattern in and of itself, becomes a skill. Because of this, the aesthetics of the technique is determined by its function and by its success. In judo, scores are awarded based solely on effectiveness and results. We don't get style points as they do in some other sports. The practical and effective application of a technique in judo is more important than what it looks like. Because of this, function dictates form. There has to be a practical and functionally efficient reason for every movement of the body when performing a skill in judo. The bottom line is that if a movement isn't practical or functional, it shouldn't be done. If a movement is done only for aesthetics, there

is no reason to perform it if you want to win on a consistent basis against skilled, fit, and resisting opponents. Shawn Watson, one of my most successful (and skillful) athletes, once remarked: "It's only pretty if it works!"

Skill Is the Practical Application of Technique

The words technique and skill are often used to mean the same thing, yet they are separate and interdependent. This part of the book is devoted to exploring what skill and technique are, and why it's important to understand how they work. Maybe to some this seems like splitting hairs, but it's my belief that to fully understand how and why judo works at a realistic, functional level, we need to put some thought, time, and effort into exploring the bio-mechanics behind the application of skilled technique against a fit, motivated, and skilled opposition. Putting it another way, how many times have we seen a great judo champion slam an opponent to the mat or secure an armlock that forces his opponent to submit? It's poetry in motion, really, and it's something even an untrained eye can appreciate. An onlooker may ask, "How did he make it look so easy?" The answer is that it took a lot of time and effort for that champion to mold that technique and make it work for him—and make it work for him against a skilled, fit, and resisting opponent. In other words, that champion made his judo work for him. As we have observed, skill is how you make a technique work for you. It cannot be said enough that skill is the practical and optimal application of technique.

Technique: A technique is a distinct movement pattern in and of itself. It's the generally accepted way of performing a throw, hold, choke, or armlock (or any movement, for that matter). Every movement the human body performs has a "technique" to it. Take walking, for example. There is a specific gait the human body has when walking efficiently. We all know what it looks like for a human being to walk normally. It is apparent when we see someone walking with a limp or an odd gait. However, there are no two human beings that have identical physical attributes and as a result there are minor (and in some cases major) variances in how each person walks. From a child's first steps, that child develops the skill necessary to walk most efficiently. While there is an accepted gait or technique for walking, everyone does it a bit differently.

Now, let's use this understanding of technique and apply it to judo. When someone thinks of o soto gari (major outer reaping throw), a specific, distinct, and finite movement comes to mind. We all recognize it as a technique where the attacker uses a forceful reaping action of one of his legs to throw his opponent. There are, however, many different ways of applying o soto gari. It's such a versatile throwing technique that it is used by people of all sizes and strength levels. All the factors involved in how the thrower actually applies the technique (and the success of his efforts) determine how skillful the whole action really is.

Each technique is different, having its own individual movement patterns, shape, form, and structure that comprise it. Seoi nage is different than okuri ashi barai. One is a forward throw with large body movements and the other is a fast-paced foot sweep. Each technique has its own function and purpose. Students should study, practice, and make every effort to master the mechanical movements of each technique—in other words, to master the basic structural movements of each technique, realizing there may be minor differences from one person to another based on body type, coordination, strength, and other factors. Once the student or athlete gains confidence and fundamental mastery of the technique (that is, the understanding of the technique's purpose and the skillful application of the structure or mechanics of the technique), he will be able to adapt it in such a way that it will become functional and work best for him.

A Technique Is a Tool

Think of a technique as a tool. How a person uses that tool is skill. A skillful application of a technique means you have used this tool in the most effective way possible under the circumstances or in a specific situation. There is more than one way to use a tool, and there is more than one way to use a technique.

This ties in with the overall concept of controlling the movement of an opponent. In other words, impose your will on your opponent as often as possible and in every possible circumstance. Make him fight on your terms, not his. This is true in both a competitive situation and in a self-defense situation. To be able to do this takes a lot of forethought, planning, and preparation. Skill in applying a technique doesn't happen overnight—it takes a lot of practice. In this instance, a throw is just like any other tool in that you have to learn how to use it and how to use it efficiently in order to get the best results from it on a consistent basis.

Some Historical Perspective

At this point, please bear with me while we take a detour into the history of judo as a sport so that the context of what we have been discussing, especially relative to the discussion of functional application of technique and skill, can be better explained.

Historically, the accepted approach to the teaching and learning of judo techniques was to learn the particular parts comprising a technique for the sake of mastering the specific movements of that particular technique. In other words, a technique was to be learned simply for the satisfaction of learning it the way it was taught in as exact of a manner as possible with no tangible alterations. Aesthetics were just as important as the practical application. Every technique had a specific "look," and any deviation or unconventional use from that was considered bad form. The student was expected to adapt his body to meet the expectations of what each particular technique looked like. A description of this approach to teaching, learning, and application could be called "process driven." In other words, the process of adapting a human body to the requirements of the technique is paramount. A person achieves satisfaction from having mastered the movement patterns that comprise the technique. The form of the technique dictates its function. While this certainly provides a great amount of satisfaction in learning and mastering a technique for the sake of learning and mastering it, it limits judo exponents in their range of exploring and mastering new technical skills. For example, for many years it was a generally accepted fact that a tall person could never really be all that good at seoi nage because he had to squat so low and his long legs prevented him from getting down so low to the mat. While the structure of seoi nage was (and is) biomechanically sound, the accepted application of what it looked like and how it was taught limited the scope and use of the technique to only those who could attain the right posture so that it would look like what a seoi nage was supposed to look like. As a result, a long-limbed person tried to perform seoi nage the same way a short-limbed person would. If your body type didn't fit seoi nage, you did something else. People with different body types were attracted to different techniques that better suited their body types. In other words, while the biomechanics of judo techniques were fundamentally correct, how people taught, learned, and applied these techniques were not practical or functional except for those whose body types best suited the mechanics of the technique.

However, it must be stressed that if the coach, student, or athlete wants to pursue a "process-driven" approach to the teaching, learning, practice, and application of techniques, that is certainly a valid choice. It's probably obvious that I am pragmatic in both theory and practice and favor the "results- or performance-driven" approach to the subject (that will be discussed in full a bit later). But this approach may not be for everyone, and the activity of judo is certainly big enough to accommodate everyone's point of view and approach to the teaching and learning of skills. In the formal, prearranged practice of any of the Kodokan judo kata, every movement is precisely established and the person's skill performing the kata is judged on how closely each technique matches the established application of that particular movement for the technique. In this case, the person performing the technique adapts his body to the structure of the technique rather than fitting the structure of the technique to his body. This is why kata is important in judo. It provides the normative structure or form of each and every technical movement in all aspects of technical application. Kata is the alphabet of judo. Each letter is shaped differently. A person must know the alphabet before he can spell a word. Kata is what "spells out" how the form or structure of a technique should be because each technique is shaped differently. From this basic technical form, variations and adaptations can be made if so desired or found to be necessary.

In the 1960s judo was growing. With the wider demographic of people wanting to participate in judo, change was inevitable. As judo became an international sporting activity, cultural and sociological changes came along with that growth. What follows are some thoughts on what effects this internationalization had on judo. The social and cultural developments in judo's history and their consequences have shaped judo's form and structure as a sport as well as a method of physical education. Consequently, when making an analysis of technical skill and movement in judo, all of this should be taken into account.

The Internationalization of Judo and Its Technical Effects

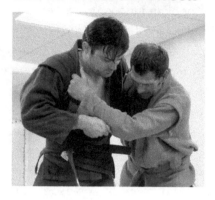

When judo grew into an international sporting activity in the 1950s and 1960s, more and more people of all body types were attracted to this new martial art. Europeans, Americans, Africans, and people of other nationalities wanted to learn judo. For the first time, an international governing body became a reality with the formation of the International Judo Federation in 1951. Judo was accepted by the International Olympic Committee as a demonstration event at the 1964 Olympic Games to be held in Tokyo, and weight classes were introduced as a requirement for its inclusion. Judo was growing, and it was about to experience some growing pains when it came to how people adapted to judo and how they made judo adapt to them.

Judo expanded throughout North and South America as well as into Europe. Japanese instructors, both affiliated and nonaffiliated with the Kodokan, were spreading Professor Kano's invention to different parts of the world during the early years of the twentieth century.

In the United States, the first generation of Japanese immigrants who learned judo in their native country brought their skills with them, settling primarily in Hawaii and on the West Coast in the early 1900s. During World War II, the Japanese-Americans in the relocation camps situated around the United States maintained their enthusiasm and practice of judo, spreading the sport to places that continue to have strong judo programs today. But it was the military servicemen stationed in Japan after World War II who learned Kodokan judo (as well as other Japanese martial arts) and brought these martial arts and their interest for them home. This was the first wave of Americans who were exposed to judo on a wide scale, and they became the instructors who introduced judo to a wider audience when they returned.

But history also tells us that it was the Europeans who made a significant impact in terms of technical development as well as organizational development on the international level outside of the Japanese. Both technical and organizational considerations were critical in the teaching and promulgation of judo, and the Europeans were effective in both. More will be said a bit later about the technical development of judo in European countries, but one major element in judo's development in Europe was that Japanese coaches in the early part of the twentieth century went to Europe to teach judo to eager European students (and technically skilled Europeans who lived and trained in Japan eventually brought their skills home with them). Strong judo programs in London, Paris, and other cities spawned national organizations and programs. All of this led to changes in technical aspects of judo as the Europeans embraced the sport but had an ability to mold it to best meet their needs.

In the Soviet Union, judo had been isolated since it had been introduced to that Communist country in the early 1900s and evolved into the Soviet hybrid of judo called sambo. What the Soviets did in isolation without the encouragement or endorsement of the Kodokan was their answer to judo. By the early 1960s, the Soviet sambo athletes who had previously been isolated from the rest of the world were competing in European judo tournaments in preparation for the 1964 Olympics, where judo would be included as a sport for the first time.

By 1938, sambo was officially recognized as a sport in the Soviet Union, attracting both members of the military and civilians. After World War II, sambo clubs sprung up all over the Soviet Union with the government's backing, and the Soviets didn't seem as interested in doing aesthetically correct techniques as much as winning. Pragmatically skillful application of a technique was paramount to these Soviet sambomen; how it looked was secondary. This approach could be described as "result or performance driven." In other words, the athlete adapts or alters the technique so it works best for him in the circumstances in which he needs it to work. The technique's function and application dictate its form.

This represented a huge shift in how people viewed the techniques of judo and the way they should be taught, practiced, and applied. Judo was no longer an exclusively Japanese martial art that Westerners wanted to emulate but was now an international sporting event. This change of viewpoint based on cultural and sociological events is important to note here. The way judo was perceived affected how it was done. A technique was no longer an end in itself; it was now a means to an end.

So when these Soviet athletes with backgrounds in sambo appeared on the international judo scene in the early 1960s with their unusual grip-fighting methods, unorthodox throws, and highly refined groundfighting skills, it sent a shockwave throughout the judo world. The Soviet sambo attitude toward judo technical skill was utilitarian, much like the similar practical view the Europeans had of judo, a view reflected in innovative technical development in all phases of judo movement and technique. In Great Britain, the Netherlands, Germany, Belgium, France, and Italy, judo had a large following, and there was certainly a no-nonsense approach to doing judo even before the Soviet sambo athletes came on the scene. An example is the great champion Anton Geesink from the Netherlands, who introduced both innovative training methods as well as new technical methods with great success. But it was the shock of the Soviet team winning four medals that most directly challenged the Japanese in their own sport in the homeland of judo in 1964 (although Geesink winning the gold medal in the "open" category of the 1964 Olympic Games certainly contributed greatly to how people looked at judo—his gold medal came as a surprise too). The significant difference was political and cultural. The Western countries maintained steady relationships with the Japanese and many of the top judo athletes trained regularly in Japan. This included the European countries as well as athletes from the United States, Canada, South America, Australia, Africa, and the Asian nations. This wasn't the case with the Soviet athletes. Generally, they were isolated from the rest of the judo world; not many people knew what to expect from them when they competed in Tokyo. The competition at the 1964 Olympics was for men only, and there were four weight classes, including the open class. The Japanese won three gold medals and the Netherlands won one. Athletes from twenty-seven nations competed, including the Soviet Union, which had four athletes entered, and all four won bronze medals. Judo was now an international sport.

So it was the Europeans and the Soviets who brought a pragmatic and functional approach into the limelight at this time. But then, didn't Kano do the same thing years before in Japan in the late nineteenth and early twentieth centuries with his eclectic and newfangled Kodokan judo? Kodokan judo has an enduring tradition of innovation, always seeking the most useful and practical approach to skill training, physical education, and character development. Jigoro Kano was considered an upstart by many in the Japanese jujutsu establishment when he started his Kodokan judo. He was an innovator. Innovation is part of judo's tradition.

Fit the Technique to the Student: A functional approach to teaching and practicing judo is to fit the technique to meet the needs of the individual performing it. It is the responsibility of a coach to teach mechanically sound, skillful, and effec-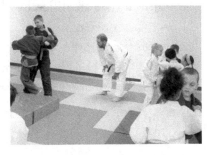tive technique to the student or athlete. A coach best serves his students by first making a thorough study of the movement he is teaching, making sure the skill is appropriate to the age and skill level, and bases what he teaches on the science of movement. Teaching a technique before students have the ability to understand it, or teaching a technique that is not based on mechanically sound principles, impedes students' ability to reach their potential.

It should be stressed again that saying the technique should fit the body does not mean that learning the fundamental technical skills is not vital. It is essential (repeat: essential) that one learns the fundamental technique correctly before adapting it to meet his or her needs. Before you can make your technique work for you, you have to know how to make the technique work in the first place! No matter how good you become, you can never stop working on your fundamentals. The throws, holds, chokes, and armlocks performed by elite judo athletes are really nothing more than fundamentals applied well and to their full potential.

Kata: The word kata means "form" or "structure." While kata has been discussed previously, for a discussion of technique to be complete, the concept of kata must be examined to see how it relates to technique and, further, how it relates to skill. Every technique has a structure. This structure determines the appearance or form of a technique and how it works biomechanically. Kata is how the technique proceeds—its primary function biomechanically. For example, a seoi nage works differently than an uchi mata. The end results are the same; they both are used to throw someone to the mat. But they are different when it comes to how they look and the way they operate in order to throw someone to the mat. Analyzing this further, the structure is what a throw looks like and the technique is the basic movement patterns of the structure. Skill is the most efficient application of the technique.

Structure: The basic form of a movement.

Technique: How the basic structure works.

Skill: Most efficient and optimal application of technique.

Is this splitting hairs? Yes it is, but if we don't split hairs and take a closer look, we'll never know the differences among these important terms.

Progression of Skill or Sequential Learning: We'll say more later about the subject of teaching technical skill and movement, but at this point it is important to say that progression is necessary for mastery of skill. The old saying "You have to walk before you can run" is certainly true. Learning takes place sequentially; one thing leads to another, and that thing leads to the next thing in a logical progression. Learn the basics, then master the basics, and then make the basics work for you. One thing really does lead to another when it comes to building new skills on top of previously learned skills. It is the coach's responsibility to see that each skill is built on previous skills in a logical progression.

Teaching **"lead-up" skills** is important in helping a student develop an optimal understanding and application of a technique. This takes time, patience, and effort on everyone's part—both students and coaches. If a student is not ready to try a specific technique, then teach movements and skills that will better direct him to learning that specific technique. As the student understands and learns one thing, he will be able to move on to the next thing. This progression of skill learning in a logical sequence ensures that the student understands why he is doing something as well as how to do it.

I've always looked at this progression in terms of adding layers to an existing technique (this will be discussed more later in this book). The coach and athlete will continue to add as many layers as necessary for the movement to be optimal. However, layers can't be added to something that's not there; mechanically fundamental elements of a technique must be mastered before layers can be added to it. As we have observed, world-class judo is essentially the fundamentals done at an optimum level of functional skill. There's no quick or easy way to develop skill. It takes time, patience, and a lot of physical and mental effort. An athlete (hopefully with the help of his coach and teammates) will eventually find a technique that "strikes a chord" or feels an affinity with. This tendency to do one technique or another is what is called "**natural frequency.**" After a new student gains the skills necessary to safely participate in randori, he will almost naturally or intuitively do one technique with more frequency than others, or in many cases move in biomechanically correct ways without ever being coached in these movements. Not every student does this, but it does take place often enough to be a noticeable effect—and certainly worth following up on as a coach. A coach can spot this simply by observing his students in randori. The frequency with which a student attempts a particular throw or groundwork technique without prompting or previous instructions from the coach is a sign of natural frequency. Some students have a natural tendency to use left-sided throwing techniques even if they were initially taught the technique on the right side. If this is the case, the coach should encourage the student to work off his left side and teach him throws from that direction from that point on. This is why it's essential for coaches to teach— and students to learn—good, solid fundamentals in all phases of judo. Along this idea of natural frequency, the coach should watch the randori sessions and take an active role in pointing out to new students what they seem to do naturally and encourage them to try those techniques more often. The coach can use this opportunity to adapt or personalize a specific technique so that it works more efficiently for the student. This type of supervised randori is one of the most beneficial activities a coach can do during a practice. Additionally, something that may not work for an athlete at an early stage of his career may work for him at a later phase of his career. As students continue to train, develop, and learn more about judo, and begin to gain mastery with their own approach to judo, they will see new aspects of the sport they never noticed before. And the reverse is true as well. That slick foot sweep an athlete used to be so good at may not be so slick after several knee operations. Being able to adapt, improvise, and overcome is part of being successful. Once we come to realize what we don't know, we progress to a higher level of learning and understanding. For real progression and mastery of skill to take place, a person must be humble enough to admit he doesn't have all the answers and, in fact, probably doesn't even know all the right questions to ask yet.

With that all said, there are some definite factors you should consider when selecting a technique to make your own. First, be honest with yourself about your strengths and weaknesses. If you don't have good explosive power or plyometric speed, you will have to choose a technique that involves some other attribute (or you can improve your explosive power so you can perform the technique better). Also, it is vital that every athlete be in excellent physical condition. As we noted earlier, elite-level judo is not possible with an unfit body. So before you select a technique to specialize in, make sure you are physically able to perform it. Not only is elite-level judo not possible to perform with an unfit body, the same is true of techniques at every level. Remember, you don't rise to the occasion. You rise to your level of training.

Second, some techniques are riskier than others. Throws like seoi nage (shoulder throw), especially the knee-drop version, and tai otoshi (body drop) are considered more stable and less risky based on the fact that both of the attacker's feet (or legs) are on the ground. Throws that come out of a slow tempo (tempo is the pace of the match, or how slow or fast the athletes are moving) are often less risky than a fast tempo throw, but then again, this isn't set in stone, so a fast-paced foot sweep just might be the safest attack to make in any given situation. Throws where you have only one foot or leg connected to the mat are considered riskier than throws that have both feet and legs on the mat. A throw like uchi mata (inner thigh throw), where one leg is supporting the attacker's body throughout the entire movement, is popular because it's so adaptable and has such a strong ballistic effect. The high impact of attacking an opponent with an uchi mata often overcomes the risk factor of attacking an opponent even though the thrower is standing on only one foot.

Third, some people are more attracted to groundfighting than to throwing or vice versa. My personal preference, ever since I was a young boy, was for newaza (groundfighting). It seemed more natural personally, and holding an opponent to the mat or forcing him to tap out was always a great source of satisfaction. As a coach, I have had many athletes over the years who were excellent at throwing and didn't share my enthusiasm for newaza. But it's my responsibility as a coach to help every athlete in my club make his judo work for him even if it's not my area of specialization.

Fourth, your physical size may have something to do with your selection of judo techniques to specialize in. The odds are that an athlete that is five feet, five inches in height and weighs 195 pounds with short legs will not tend to favor a technique like sankaku jime (triangle choke) due to the fact that it is really hard to form a triangle around an opponent's neck and arm with such short legs. However, that short, stocky athlete may have a terrific uchi mata, using it just as well as a tall, lanky athlete who also uses uchi mata. Uchi mata is such a versatile and adaptable technique that each of these athletes may adapt and modify the throw to suit the needs of his individual body type. The short athlete's uchi mata won't look like the tall athlete's uchi mata, but it will still be an uchi mata and will be successful for each athlete in his own way.

A Thorough Study of Fundamentals Is Essential

There are other factors in determining what technique works best for an athlete in any given situation, but by far the best way to find out is to make a thorough study of good fundamentals, drill on them consistently, and then do as much randori as possible to find out what works best through trial and error. The only way students will be able to find out what works best for them is to study and learn as many techniques as possible. If someone has never tried a technique, he will never know if it will work for him. The old saying "You will never succeed until you try" is certainly true.

Students should enter as many club, local, and regional judo tournaments as possible early in their careers and try things out after they have gained technical skill in ukemi (falling techniques) and some basic techniques involving both standing and ground-fighting. It's also important to engage in as much randori as possible. Randori should always be supervised by the coach and should have a purpose. Randori is not a tournament—it is training. There are no "winners" or "losers" in randori. It is also a great place to find out if you need more work on something. Don't ever hesitate to try a new technique, especially in randori. That's the best way to really find out what works best for you. From these experiences in randori and in local tournaments, athletes can refine their technical skills so that it starts to have a higher rate of success.

Rate of Success: Just because a technique is complicated does not necessarily mean it is effective. The more efficiently you apply a technique, the higher the rate of success. If you can do a move in two steps instead of three and still make it work on a regular, consistent basis 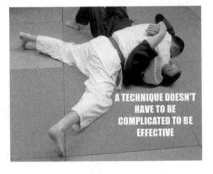 with a high rate of success, then good for you (and bad for your opponent). A good opponent won't wait for you to throw him or slap an armlock on him; you have to perform the technique in the most efficient and quickest way possible. Be efficient and economical in your movement. Another way of saying this is to take your time, but do it in a hurry.

A technical skill that works reliably and effectively in a variety of situations is the go-to move for an athlete—his **tokui waza** (tokui translates to "specialty" and waza translates to "technique"). An athlete might have more than one tokui waza, depending on the circumstance. Other athletes might have one specialty technique they seem to catch everyone with. If an athlete uses a specific technique often that results in a score or ippon, that skill has a high ratio of success. This also relates to using the right movement or technique at the right time during a match. An athlete may have a specific technique or movement he uses in a specific situation with good results and he knows he can usually count on it when he needs it. This move has a high rate of success in that specific situation. This is similar to a tokui waza, or favorite technique, but applied in a more tactical way. In any event, one of the benchmarks of an effective technical skill is its rate of success. Conversely, if an athlete thinks his tokui waza is something that never seems to work for him, but he just likes doing it in practice, he should definitely rethink this and choose a technique that has a higher rate of success in an actual situation during randori or a during a match.

World sambo champion Maurice Allan gave me some great advice in 1976: "Make the technique work for you." Here are some questions to ask yourself to determine if your judo works for you.

1. Can you perform the technique automatically? Is it there for you when you need it?

2. Does it have a high ratio of success? Is it reliable?

3. Does it work against opponents who are competitive or have the same skill level as you? Does it work on resisting, fit, and skilled opponents?

4. Do you enjoy doing it? Does it feel right when you perform it? There is an old saying that "you should feel your judo." In other words, there is a kinesthetic awareness that everything

is working as it should. This describes the sweet spot, or **debana** (instant of opportunity)—that moment when the timing is perfect and the technique is working optimally.

5. Is it versatile? Can you use it in more than one situation?

In other words, training should and must be balanced so the athlete has the strength, endurance, functional technical ability, and mental/emotional capacity to be successful. Athletes who lack in any of these areas will not reach their potential. It bears repeating that it is the coach's job (as well as the athlete's job—after all, it's the athlete who is doing it) to train so the athlete has the most functional power available to him. In other words, the athlete must train to increase his power. An athlete must know how (and be able) to apply his power to the technique. The athlete uses the movement of his body to create the momentum and control necessary for a successful attack. In this way, the athlete literally makes his body part of the technique. This is in keeping with what Professor Kano meant when he said, "The maximum-efficient use of mind and body is the fundamental principle governing all the techniques of judo." The phrase "maximum-efficient" directly implies that technical skill is more easily and more effectively achieved if athletes use their physical and mental attributes in the most efficient way possible. In real terms, this translates to economy and efficacy of movement when applying a technique. To best achieve this, an athlete's body must have the physical capacity to work at this level of efficiency. The athlete must develop skill with the technique so it works best for him based on both his physical attributes and limitations. This is why we come to practice. It takes a lot of time and effort to achieve functional skill. For the technique to be effective, the mechanics of it must work best for the person doing it.

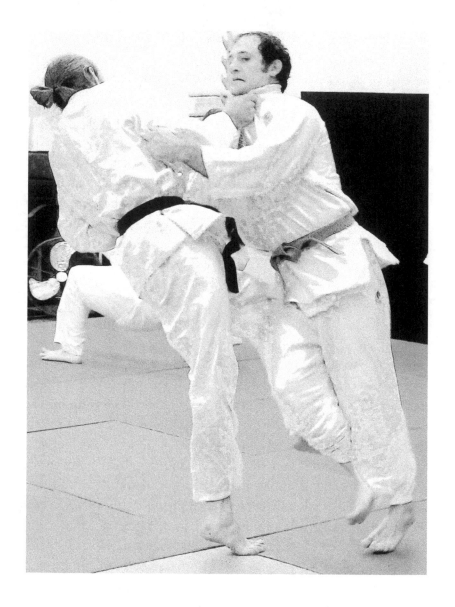

"Kuzushi is the description for the sum total of movement."
—James Bregman

CHAPTER 3

Controlling Movement: Kuzushi

Controlling Movement: Kuzushi

Controlling movement is a difficult skill to learn and master. Two important factors are that you must 1. control your own body posture, balance, stance, footwork, and movement; 2. control your opponent's posture, balance, stance, footwork, and movement. Controlling your own body movement is difficult enough, but in judo, we are required to control the body movement of an opponent (who is often resisting) as well.

Kuzushi: Without It, Judo Is Not Possible

As we discussed in the previous chapter, the underlying principle of judo is "ju." The physical application of ju is kuzushi. Essentially, kuzushi and controlling movement are one in the same. Most every judo student knows that kuzushi is one of the primary elements that comprise a throwing technique. Kuzushi is almost taken for granted, and probably because of that, not enough time is spent on mastering it. In judo circles it is often said that "kuzushi is movement" or "without movement, there is no kuzushi." This chapter explains the biomechanical reasons behind why kuzushi works. Let's start with the two primary methods of controlling movement and balance.

Happo no Kuzushi: Eight Directions of Breaking Balance

The first method of controlling movement and balance is happo no kuzushi ("happo" means "eight directions," "no" means "of," and "kuzushi" implies the breaking of balance). It is the method most judo students spend time studying. Happo no kuzushi are the eight directions in which balance can be broken:

1. Front
2. Back
3. Right side
4. Left side
5. Right front corner
6. Right rear corner
7. Left front corner
8. Left rear corner

In kuzushi, the attacker transmits direct force against the opponent's weak areas of balance. This is a direct means of controlling an opponent's movement. The attacker initiates power and uses the direct velocity (speed and direction of movement) to control his opponent. These eight directions of controlling balance and movement provide a basic framework for the understanding of throwing techniques.

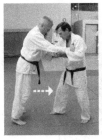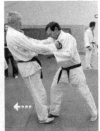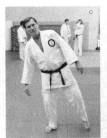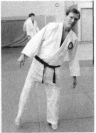

The four sides of controlling kuzushi (photos left to right): 1. front, 2. back, 3. right, 4. left.

Four Sides and Four Corners: From a mechanical point of view, there are four sides and four corners comprising eight different angles in the application of happo no kuzushi. The four sides are front, back, right side, and left side. The four corners are front right, front left, rear right, and rear left. Consider the human body as a wheel. The center of the body (or wheel) is the axis (like a hub in a wheel). The axis extends from the

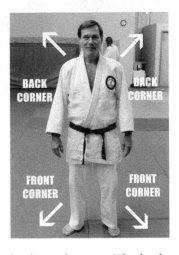

top of the head down the middle of the body to the mat. The body moves and turns around this axis like a wheel moves around its hub. When the body moves (or is moved by another body), it will go into the direction of one of these eight angles. While it is entirely possible to break someone's balance when he is standing still (sometimes, an athlete will catch his opponent "flat-footed" and take advantage of the situation by throwing him), using movement will exponentially increase the possibility of success in applying a throwing technique by controlling an opponent with body movement.

Kuzushi Controls the Opponent's Stability: Balance is dependent upon the stability of the body. When standing in shizentai (natural upright posture), the feet should extend in a line down from the hips. This provides stability and permits optimal mobility

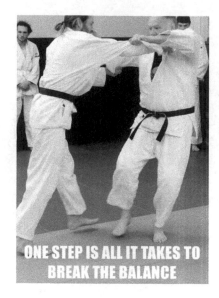

ONE STEP IS ALL IT TAKES TO BREAK THE BALANCE

for the athlete. A stance that is too narrow or too wide does not provide for adequate stability and mobility. The weight distribution on both feet should be equal. The feet are important, as the athlete should place his weight primarily on the front part of his foot and toes. The toes are important in maintaining balance and stability.

If an opponent stands still, the attacker's best option is to break his opponent's balance forward or backward in a direction vertical to a straight line going through the opponent's feet. If an opponent is moving, it is most efficient to pull or push him in the direction he is moving. The attacker uses his whole body to move and control his opponent and does not simply rely on pushing or pulling with his hands. If the attacker pulls or pushes with the same amount of force with which the defender resists, posture and balance won't be broken. The pulling or pushing action of the attacker must be greater than his opponent's, and the most effective way to do that is to move the opponent. Movement provides controlled motion and greatly assists the attacker in generating more force into the pulling or pushing action. The attacker moves his opponent's body, pulling or pushing it with force generated from his own body (starting with his lower extremities and moving through his hips and body), and the force is transferred to his hands at the point of contact with the opponent. The combination of his own movement along with his opponent's greatly enhances the action of kuzushi. The velocity generated by both the attacker's and defender's moving bodies increases the force generated by the attacker in applying the throw.

Happo no kuzushi is direct in its intent but subtle in its application. An opponent is often simply moved into the direction of one of the angles. Even if an opponent takes just one step, that is all that is required to take control of his balance and throw him. In the staccato pace of a judo match, the athletes accelerate, decelerate, and change directions the entire time. This type of movement is ideal for initiating an attack. If the attacker pulls at the optimal instant (debana, or instant of opportunity), the opponent's balance will be broken. Movement is the prime factor in controlling an opponent's balance. However, in many cases, an athlete will use hando no kuzushi, the second method of controlling movement and balance, to elicit a reaction from an opponent.

Hando no Kuzushi: Reaction Forms of Breaking Balance

In this second method of controlling and breaking balance, the attacker acts using direct power and then uses his opponent's reaction to attack him with a throw. The best way to explain this is that you push, he pushes back, and you pull. Every action causes an equal and opposite reaction. You push and your opponent resists by pulling away; you pull and your opponent pushes. Just about every sport has some type of "action-reaction" movement, and in an activity like judo, where balance is a key to victory, it is considered essential. Basically, an opponent unbalances himself by reacting to the attacker's initial movement (such as a feint or diversionary attack). There will be more on this when renzoku waza (continuation techniques) and renraku waza (combination techniques) are discussed later in this part of the book.

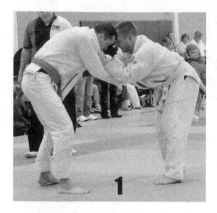

1. Here is an example of using hando no kuzushi in a practical application. In this tomoe nage photo sequence, the attacker pulls down as he pushes his opponent in order to get the opponent to resist.

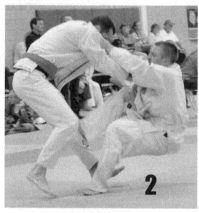

2. The opponent took the bait and made one step forward as he pushed back on the attacker. The attacker took advantage of this, stepped in, and swung under his opponent to start the tomoe nage.

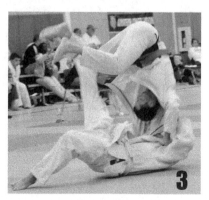

3. The opponent literally walked into the tomoe nage and was thrown for ippon. (In a discussion with me after the match, the athlete who threw his opponent with this tomoe nage told me he "tested" his opponent once earlier in the match to see how his opponent would react. He learned that this opponent had no lateral movement and would react to a push by pushing back forcefully. This tactical application of hando no kuzushi proved effective and scored ippon.)

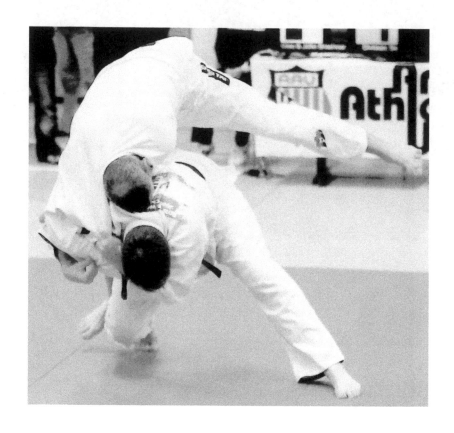

"Everything is a handle."

—Rene Pommerelle

CHAPTER 4

Controlling and Breaking Posture

Controlling and Breaking an Opponent's Posture

Though posture plays a key role in every sport, it is an integral part of judo because it so directly is affected by the use of kuzushi. Having said this, please read the preceding chapter on Kuzushi, as everything that is discussed in that chapter directly relates to what is in this chapter. An integral part of kuzushi is controlling an opponent's posture: break his posture and you break his balance. Having and using the optimal posture permits allows for a technically more effective application in any sport. Let's take a look at how, in judo, posture is a vital link in controlling one's own movement and balance as well as in controlling an opponent's movement and balance.

Shisei: Posture

The actual structure of how a human body presents itself is "posture," which is called **shisei** (meaning posture, and generally used in judo to also imply stance). The posture of the body and the stance (or position) of the feet are factors that determine the efficiency of footwork and body movement as well as the transfer of power from the feet up through the body and into the action of a throw. Optimal posture is necessary for an athlete to have freedom of movement. An optimal posture is relatively straight and upright, where the spine is not bent or curved forward. A curved spine limits movement and inhibits transfer of power in attacking. The shoulders should ideally be in a line extending from the hips—in other words, each shoulder should be over each hip and the hips should ideally be in line with the feet. If the athlete's feet are too far apart or too close to each other, they provide less stability than well-positioned feet. An athlete who is bent over with a rounded spine places too much weight on his feet as he steps. This is what is called "heavy feet." These heavy feet are being used by the athlete to stabilize his poorly distributed body weight in an effort to provide better balance for himself, which means he is not using his feet to create movement. Posture and stance are fundamentally important to the freedom of movement and, ultimately, to the generation of the force necessary for attacking an opponent.

An effective posture is one that permits the athlete to be ready to transfer the energy from his body into the body of his unsuspecting opponent at any time. In some striking sports, this is the "ready stance," where the athlete is not relaxed but not tense, like a spring ready to unleash its energy. An effective posture and stance permit the athlete to always be ready to move as necessary. It also serves as the power chain in transferring force from the feet into the attack.

The two primary postures in judo are **shizentai** (natural posture) and **jigotai** (defensive posture). Both have their uses and both have different applications and variations, but these two postural positions provide a basic framework for the study and use of posture.

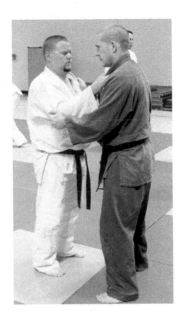

Shizentai: Meaning "natural posture," this is an upright posture allowing athletes the most freedom of movement and control of their own bodies. In shizentai, when the two athletes are gripping each other, the distance between the hips of the athletes is usually a bit more than the length of a hand (but can be closer or farther in proximity depending on the situation). This allows for freedom of movement, and the hips are close enough to attack and defend freely. The back is straight but not rigid. The shoulders are not hunched forward and the weight of the athlete's body is distributed evenly. The feet are positioned in a straight line extending down from the hips to afford maximum balance, allowing for efficient foot movement. This upright posture's main structural support is the spine. Much like a beam in a building, the spine serves to provide stability and support for the human body. An upright posture permits the transference of power up through the body that is generated by the feet in launching a throwing attack. The feet, driving off the mat, generate force that is transmitted up through the legs into the hips and torso of the attacker and up and through the shoulders, arms, and hands to its final transfer into the opponent's body. This power chain is exactly that, a chain, and to transfer power along its length, a chain must be straight with no kinks if it is to work efficiently. Shizentai is the ideal posture to use when attempting to throw an opponent. There are as many variations of shizentai as there are people using it, but the reason shizentai works is because of a straight (not rigid) spine that allows for the body to be upright and well balanced.

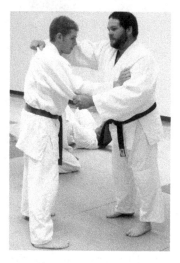

Novices may think that the structural posture of shizentai requires that they use only the basic kumi kata method of holding the lapel and sleeve. But any method of gripping can be used when using shizentai. While the grip and posture are linked, there is a huge variety of gripping methods used in judo and sambo, and a strong, upright posture allows the athlete to move with more stability and freedom when choosing and using a grip.

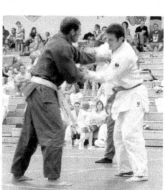

This photo shows how shizentai is used for optimal control in distribution of body weight as the athletes move within range of each other and are about to engage in grip fighting. The athlete on the left has good weight distribution in his feet and leads with his right foot and leg as he extends his left hand and arm out to get his initial grip. This is optimal distribution of his body weight as he leads with his right foot and leg as he extends his left hand and arm out. If he had led with his left foot and leg as he reached out with his left hand and arm, he would have been vulnerable to a foot sweep or other throw, as the weight distribution would have been off balance.

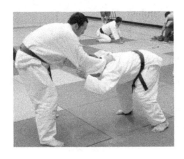

Jigotai: This is called defensive or bent-over posture. While both athletes in this photo are in jigotai, the one on the right is at an extremely defensive posture. In jigotai, the athlete believes that by bending over and keeping his hips at a far distance from his opponent, he is safe from a throwing attack. In reality, the athlete's posture is broken with his shoulders and head too far in front of his hips, putting him off balance and vulnerable. From this position, the athlete is not in a strong position to launch an effective throwing attack or provide an effective defense against an opponent's attack. Structurally, the curved spine inhibits power generated by the feet in a throwing attack from being directed through the body. This curved spine is like a sharp turn in the road for a speeding car, slowing it down. Additionally, the distribution of the body's weight is off balance, with the athlete's head and shoulders far forward and in front of his hips and feet.

The photo used here shows two types of jigotai. The athlete on the left is in more of a "classic" defensive posture with feet wide and a curved back hunching forward with lowered head. His upper body, shoulders, and head are forward and in front of his hips. He is placing weight in his buttocks and hips in an effort to crouch deeper to make space between himself and his opponent as well as to avoid being pulled forward. The athlete on the right is, again, in an extremely defensive position, and while his spine is straight, his head, shoulders, and upper body are far forward and in front of his hips. His feet are in a wide stance. He is using his hands and arms to pull down on his opponent as he backs away with the intention of moving away and out of danger. The primary goal of jigotai is to stall and should obviously be considered passive or "negative" judo. This defensive position, when most effectively used, is temporary only and used with the intent of creating as much space as possible between the defender's hips and the attacker's hips. Jigotai is a natural defensive posture; to avoid being thrown, you automatically want to curl in and get as low and as close to the ground as possible. Much like a baby in the womb in the fetal position, the body goes into this almost-fetal, curled, bent-over posture when in danger.

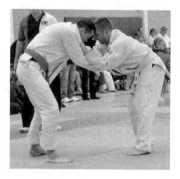

However, being crouched is not always a defensive posture. Some athletes prefer the low, crouching posture in order to create some space between the attacker's body and his opponent's body as a method of slowing down the pace of the match, to gain more distance to enter into an attack, or to elicit a reaction from the opponent as part of hando no kuzushi (breaking balance by opponent's reaction) to open a body gap as a setup for a throwing attack. In this photo, the attacker on the right momentarily leaned forward in a crouching position and pulled his opponent down as he pushed him to get the opponent to push back and step forward. The attacker then hit in with a tomoe nage for the ippon. In looking at the crouched position of the two athletes in this photo, the attacker on the right is crouched and bending at the waist, but the noticeable difference is that his spine is straight. This straight spine allows the force generated from his feet to be transmitted more efficiently through his body when he launches his throwing attack. The athlete on the left is bent over with a curved spine in a typical example of jigotai. It is clear that this athlete is defensive and does not want to engage with his opponent.

Posture and Hips Are Linked Together: Posture is important in exerting control over an opponent because of the importance of the hips in initiating force and velocity in movement. An upright posture allows the hips to be closer to the opponent, and because of the upright posture, the hips can better be brought into use, both offensively and defensively. My old friend Harry Parker once said, "Lead with your hips." (More on this a bit later in the analysis of the "lead

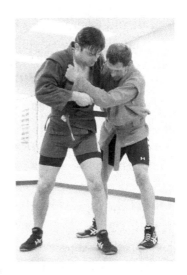

leg.") By doing this, an athlete can attack and defend with greater accuracy—but to be successful, it is essential to have a good, upright posture. Additionally, the bent-over posture places the shoulders out in front of the hips, making the athlete unbalanced in the front. This posture also places a majority of weight in the athlete's buttocks, making him vulnerable to the rear as well. The bent-over posture also naturally forces what are called "heavy feet," where the athlete generates too much downward force pushing into the mat with his feet. This prevents the athlete from moving freely to generate velocity or pivot quickly enough. The bent-over posture, moreover, creates what is called "giving your opponent your hips." In other words, this bent-over posture allows the opponent the space to initiate an attack with greater force and to get under the bent-over athlete's center of gravity more easily. This is why posture is fundamentally important to teach to students. Without good posture, power (resulting in the application of good skill in technique) cannot be sufficiently applied.

Stance: Be positioned in the right place at the right time. Foot placement and how an athlete stands, combined with his posture, are referred to as "stance." Stance is an integral part of posture. The concept of shisei combines both posture and stance—how a person stands and where he stands. **Tachi** is translated as "to stand" and also implies how a person stands, and **tachi-ai** translates to "meet together for combat." So for general purposes these terms refer to "stance" as used in the martial arts (although the term shisei is often used generically to include both posture and stance in judo). The foot position an athlete has at the start of his attack is crucial in the efficient application and execution of the movement pattern he wants to use. I have often told my students, "If you start in the wrong place, you will end up in the wrong place." One of the biggest hurdles novices face in learning how to throw is their stance at the start of the throwing movement. There are two primary stances used in judo, with many variations based on necessity or opportunity. These basic stances are ai yotsu and kenka yotsu.

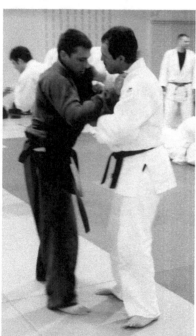

Ai Yotsu: Same-Side Stance

This situation occurs when both athletes lead with the same-side hip and foot; in other words, a righty versus a righty. This situation is common and is often ideal when learning new technical skills as it can be used as a neutral position. Any method of gripping can be used, and ai yotsu takes place in both shizentai and jigotai situations. The predominant feature of this stance is that both athletes lead with the same hip, leg, and foot.

Kenka Yotsu: Opposite-Side Stance

This happens when one athlete leads with his right side and his opponent leads with his left side. In this situation, there is often more space between the athletes, but this may not always be the case. Both shizentai and jigotai postures are used in kenka yotsu. The main feature of this stance is that the athletes lead

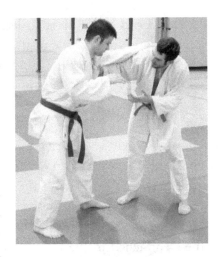

with the opposite hip, leg, and foot. In kenka yotsu situations, each athlete attempts to gain the dominant control of grip, posture, and stance. Each will then attempt to get the "inside hip" in order to more effectively attack the opponent.

Get the Inside Hip

Often when in a kenka yotsu situation, the athlete who manages to get his hip in front of his opponent's hip will be better able to sneak in an attack. As shown in this photo, the athlete on the right has managed to get his right hip on the "inside" or in front of his opponent's left hip. This affords him an ideal position to attack with his seoi nage. Any throw can be used,

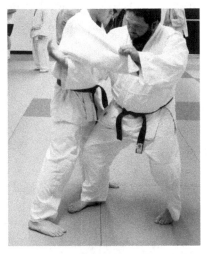

but having the inside hip permits closer proximity to the axis of the opponent's body. If an athlete gets the inside hip position, he will also have the "inside foot," which permits him to launch reaping leg attacks such as o uchi gari or ko uchi gari.

The "Lead Leg": Most athletes will lead with an extended hip, leg, and foot on one side or the other when they compete. This is often called the "lead leg," but in reality the hip is what is leading with the leg and foot positioned under it. As illustrated in the photos showing ai yotsu, one athlete will lead with his right foot, leg, and hip, and his opponent will do the same. In kenka yotsu, one athlete will lead with his left foot, leg, and hip, and his opponent will lead with his right foot, leg, and hip. In either case, the athletes have a "lead leg" in the same way a boxer will use a lead leg in his boxing stance. What actually occurs is that the athlete will lead with one hip or the other, and as we saw before, the leg and foot (being attached to the hip) will be positioned under the lead hip. This is actually what is meant by the common piece of advice, "**Lead with your hips**." By leading with a hip, an athlete will be far less likely to extend his leg or foot too far out in front, making for an easy target for the opponent to attack. Making sure that the leg and foot are positioned directly under the hip, the athlete will attain a more stable and balanced stance.

Leading with the hips provides more efficient and powerful rotational movement positioned on a stable base when attacking or defending. In some cases, an athlete will extend his foot or leg as "bait" for his opponent to attack. This is called a "**sugar foot**" in wrestling and is an applicable term in judo as well. This implies that attacking the extended foot is too sweet of an opportunity for an opponent to pass up. But this sugar foot has been put out there to lure the opponent into the attack only to be countered by the athlete who offered the sugar foot as bait.

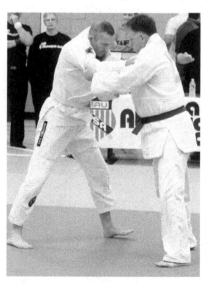

However, some athletes will not lead with either hip or leg and foot and will work out of a "**square stance**" similar to the isosceles stance used in shooting. In this stance, the athlete does not advance hip, leg, or foot and squarely faces his opponent. This photo shows the athlete on the right using a square stance as his opponent on the left starts to step forward with his left foot as they engage in grip fighting. Regardless of the grip the athlete uses, this square stance can provide a mechanically stable base. From my experience and research, the square stance is most often used by athletes who are counter fighters who wait for the opponent to make the initial move in order to counter it with their own attack.

Newaza Shisei: This means "posture in groundfighting." The role of effective posture is not limited to using and applying throwing techniques from a standing position. Posture is equally important in groundfighting. While we most often think of the posture of the human body in standing situations, the posture in newaza is equally important. The same biomechanical principles 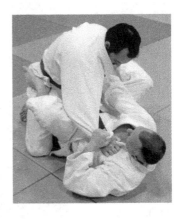 apply to posture in groundfighting as in standing. This is because posture is the structural position of the human body. However, in standing situations, the posture can change more freely than in groundfighting. This is primarily because the base points on the mat (the parts of the body actually touching the mat) are greater in newaza than in standing. In standing, the feet are what touch the mat but in groundfighting, there are more points touching the mat. This increased number of such points makes it harder to move. While there is more stability in groundfighting because of the larger and more stable base area, there is less freedom of movement. With less mobility in newaza, groundfighting positions are held for a longer period of time, and controlling the position of the opponent plays a larger role than it does in standing judo. The primary purpose of posture in groundfighting is to control the position of the opponent and gain a superior position. An athlete's goal is to constantly attempt to control the opponent's position and improve his own position until he is able to secure a scoring move.

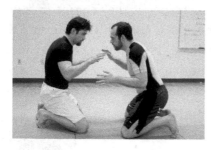

This photo shows a basic neutral groundfighting position. The posture is upright with the weight distribution evenly spaced on the knees and feet serving as the base. The head is upright and not positioned too far ahead of the hips. This newaza position affords the athletes as much freedom of movement as possible.

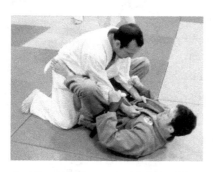

Newaza no Semekata: Meaning "forms of attack in groundfighting," the most basic position used for many years in Kodokan judo is this supine or recumbent position. Newaza translates to "reclining or supine" technique. What is now called the "guard" is one of the oldest positions used in judo. Sumiyuki Kotani, Yoshimi Osawa, and Yuichi Hirose made specific reference to newaza no semekata (attacking forms of supine techniques) in their book *Newaza of Judo* published in 1973. This name describes the tactical and technical purpose of this position as primarily an offensive position. While defensive skills were initiated from this position, the intent was to attack. There is a wide variety of movement used in newaza. The Western concept of wrestling where a pin fall is scored and the wrestler loses when his shoulders touch the mat simultaneously was never a consideration for the early Japanese judo exponents. Fighting from the buttocks, hips, or back is simply another position that can be used to take advantage of an opponent. Some of the exponents of the Kosen judo movement in Japanese schools starting in the early twentieth century turned this position into a science and an art, making it one of their primary fighting positions. This newaza position was a primary groundfighting position taught by Mitsuo Maeda to the early proponents of what was to develop into Brazilian jiu-jitsu in the 1920s in Brazil. The centrality of this position in Brazilian jiu-jitsu is well known and in many ways similar to how it is taught and used by Kosen judo exponents. The phrase "newaza" has been used generically for many years in judo to describe groundwork in general. This is most likely because this position was the primary posture used in groundfighting from judo's inception.

Rides: The purpose of a ride is to control the opponent for as long as necessary in order to apply a submission technique or pin. As judo became an international sport, groundfighting tactics and technical skills were altered in the same way standing judo's tactics and technical skills were. Certainly one signifi-

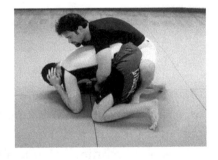

cant change tactically and technically since the 1960s and 1970s was the increased adoption of wrestling positions and technical skills in judo. This photo shows a basic application of the spiral ride. The basic idea behind a ride in judo is similar to wrestling— controlling an opponent to gain time, allowing the attacker more opportunity to improve his position and break the defender down in order to apply a pin or submission technique. However, in judo, we don't get points for riding an opponent as is done in wrestling, and as a result rides have been altered and adapted to better suit the tactical and technical requirements of judo.

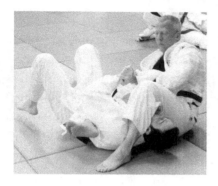

In a very real sense, any method of controlling an opponent in groundfighting can be considered a "ride." Controlling an opponent in a **leg press** as shown in this photo is essentially a ride because the attacker exerts control over his opponent for a period of time, allowing him increased opportunities to secure a scoring technique.

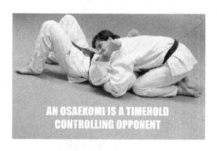

AN OSAEKOMI IS A TIMEHOLD CONTROLLING OPPONENT

Timehold: Holding and controlling an opponent in osaekomi waza for a specified period of time is a "timehold." Gene LeBell first used this term, as far as I know, back in the 1960s. A timehold has two primary purposes: 1. to hold and control the opponent long enough to score points or be awarded ippon, and 2. to hold and control the opponent for as long as necessary with the intention of applying a submission technique or finishing hold. This twofold purpose is the basic definition of **osaekomi waza** (pinning or immobilization techniques). An osaekomi waza is not a "pin" the same way a pin is used in wrestling with the goal of pinning the shoulders on the mat. So, in very real terms, osaekomi waza is a timehold.

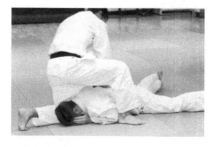

Position is a term that has been used often in this book and refers to: 1. where an object (in our case, an athlete's body) is in relation to its environment or surroundings (for our purposes, the location on the mat), and 2. its relation to other objects or bodies in the same location at the same time. In other words, where an athlete's body is at any given time on the mat and where he is relative to his opponent at any given time. Most people think of "position" primarily in groundfighting, but position is certainly a factor in standing work as well. The popular saying, "control the position and get the submission" certainly is true. What an athlete does when he controls the position is to control his opponent's movement. This photo shows the bottom athlete in one of the worst positions possible and that is flat on his front in the utsubuse (hiding or facedown) position. An athlete waiting for the referee to call "matte" to get out of trouble is not always the best tactic and often permits an opponent to take advantage of the situation.

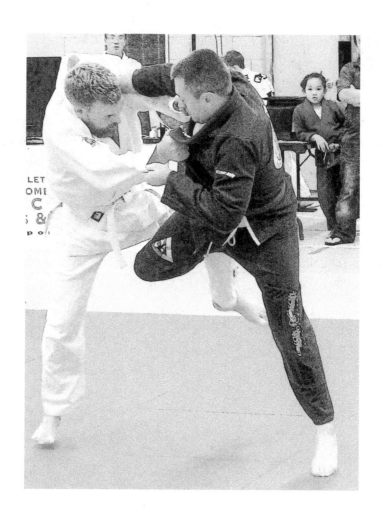

"You have to play a long time to be able to play like yourself."
—Miles Davis

CHAPTER 5

Applying Technical Skill

Applying Technical Skill: Kuzushi, Tsukuri, Kake, and Kime

This is the series of actions that are the primary building blocks of every technical skill, both in throwing and in groundfighting. These are kuzushi, tsukuri, kake, and—although unofficial in terms of Kodokan judo's approach to the subject—kime. These actions of kuzushi, tsukuri, kake, and kime are sequential, building on each other in a progression of movement phases. One thing must happen before the next thing starts, and if that first thing isn't done optimally, the second thing won't happen. While most people think of these steps or building blocks only in terms of throwing techniques, they are just as relevant for the techniques of groundfighting.

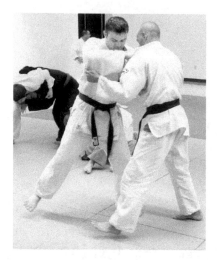

Kuzushi: The word kuzushi implies breaking of balance and posture. Kuzushi is an important concept in the study, practice, application, and teaching of judo. The concept of controlling the movement of an opponent and the ultimate breaking of his posture, stance, or balance is what makes all judo techniques efficient in their application. The action that starts the process of kuzushi is force, which the attacker uses to initiate movement. This is different than simple brute force, however. Functional application of strength is what is necessary. The attacker focuses his strength on an opponent's vulnerable point. No matter what anyone says, the use of force is based on optimal physical strength and fitness. A strong, fit athlete always has a huge advantage over an athlete who is physically unprepared or weak. It must be stressed that effective kuzushi is dependent on controlling the defender's movement. The power generated by the attacker creates the movement necessary to break or control the defender's movement, balance, posture, and stance. If insufficient force is generated, the defender's body will not be moved, and kuzushi will not occur. In other words, movement is the key factor in effective kuzushi. The better you control movement, the more effective your skill will be. Kuzushi directly implies a "breaking down" of the opponent's posture, balance, and stance.

Kuzushi can be divided into two distinct, sequential parts. First, the attacker actually moves his opponent, even if it is only to move him one step. That movement entails direction, so the attacker must move his opponent into a specific direction. The tempo or pace with which the attacker moves his opponent is a key element in the success of that movement. A good example is that it is mechanically impossible to step slowly and successfully perform okuri ashi barai (sliding foot sweep). This technique's success relies on velocity (speed and directional control), which comes from a fast tempo. Another element of this first part is that to successfully force an opponent to move, the attacker must generate enough force to make his opponent move away from his initial stance. The stance is simply how an athlete stands: how far his feet are apart; which hip, leg, or foot he leads with; where his weight distribution is; and what his initial posture is (upright or crouched). Once the attacker gets his opponent to move from the opponent's initial stance, the second part of kuzushi is ready to come into play, which is for the attacker to control the posture of his opponent. By moving the opponent's body, the attacker will control or "break" his opponent's posture. In much the same way an earthquake crumbles the foundation of a building, the initial movement and taking an opponent away from his stance cause the breaking down of the structure of the opponent's posture. When the opponent's posture breaks, his weight distribution becomes unbalanced and he is susceptible to being immediately set up for a seamless transition to tsukuri.

Tsukuri: This word implies "building," "constructing," or "forming" a technique. Tsukuri is often explained in terms of fitting or placing the body in position in order to apply the technique. The tsukuri action flows smoothly from kuzushi, so much so that it is hard to tell them apart if done optimally. This is the point where the attacker uses the speed of his action and the direction of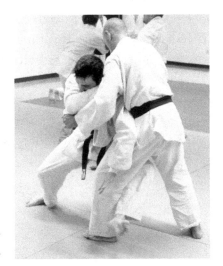

his movement to direct both how his body moves and how the defender's body moves. It is the point where the attacker starts to develop or form the specific technique she intends to use. This "building" of the technique relies on the kinetic energy generated in the kuzushi action using the inertia of the defender's body movement. It is in this tsukuri phase that the attacker's mechanically correct placement and use of his feet, legs, hands, legs, and head makes the technique successful. The attacker must put the right body part in the right place at the right time for the tsukuri or construction of the technique to be accomplished. The great basketball coach John Wooden said, "Small things make big things happen." This describes what takes place in tsukuri. Knowing why and when an arm has to move a certain way at the exact time it needs to move is what is meant by "small things." Every technique is composed of different individual parts or movements, and the tsukuri phase is where these parts have to come together like parts of a puzzle. Once these parts come together and create or build the structure of the technique, the attacker transitions into the next phase of the throwing action, and that is kake—actually getting the opponent into the air.

An important part of tsukuri is the fact that the attacker and defender are no longer two independent bodies but are now joined together as one unit. This unit is a **couple**. The attacker attaches his body to the defender's body and builds his technique on this attachment. This is what is meant when it is said that the technique is "built" or "formed" in this tsukuri action. **Coupling** is the connection of two parts (in this case, the attacker and defender's bodies) in such a way that they work together as one unit.

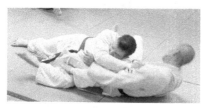

Kake: This is the actual throwing action of the attack. Kake can be translated as "suspend" and specifically refers to taking the opponent from his feet and putting him in the air, suspending and controlling his body in the process. This is the peak or apex of the throw. At this point, the attacker has the best control of the defender's body he will have in the entire action. This is the moment of the most impact between the attacker and defender's bodies with maximum power generated by the attacker. If this were a punch from a boxer, it would be the instant the boxer's fist hits the opponent's jaw or body. This is the execution of the technique that is the result of the kuzushi and tsukuri actions. An integral aspect of kake is the attacker and defender holding onto each other. Recall that this is called a "couple." The movement of the attacker's action in applying the technique is amplified by the defender being thrown. In other words, by the attacker falling, the attacker's throwing action (either the push or a pull that initiated the action) is enhanced because now the attacker and defender are attached together as a couple. The gravitational pull of the two bodies is greater on just one. As a result of this coupling, the velocity is greatly accelerated and a greater ballistic effect is achieved.

Biomechanically, kake can be divided into two sequential parts: 1. initial lift and 2. trajectory control. This may sound like a description of a rocket's flight, but the same principles can be used for a human body going through the air as much as for a rocket. In this first part, the attacker's ballistic execution of the throw physically lifts the opponent and projects him off the mat. Depending on the throwing movement, the direction of the initial lifting action will differ. In other words, the lift will look different when doing okuri ashi barai than when doing uchi mata. In each instance, the defender is lifted off the mat, but the direction is different due to the different functions of each throw. This initial explosive lifting action transitions to the second part of kake, and that is the control of the movement of the defender. How the defender moves through the air is "flight" or "trajectory" in the same way a rocket moves through the air; and just as a rocket lifting off the launch pad has to be guided in its flight, the human body is lifted off the mat and is guided or controlled by the attacker performing the technique. The more efficiently the attacker controls his opponent's body movement while the opponent is in the air, the better control the attacker will have in landing him on the mat. This trajectory control starts with the defender leaving the mat from a standing position and ends with the defender landing on the mat on his back or backside. This sequence of action transitions into kime.

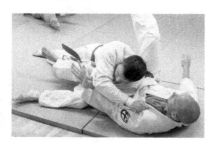

Kime: This can be translated as "to finish" or "to decide." The term **zanshin** is also used to describe this finishing action of a throw. The word zanshin refers to "awareness" with the purpose of not relaxing but remaining focused in the final execution of a throwing technique. This is a sound concept, but I believe kime is more direct and equally sound in its concept in describing what happens at the finish of a throwing technique, so I will use this term. While not one of Kodokan judo's three constructs or building blocks of a technique, think of kime as the follow-through or finish to the technique. This is the action that ensures the termination of the sequence of actions that make up the technique. Think of a batter in baseball who swings his bat and follows through with his swing. Once the bat makes contact with the baseball, the batter doesn't stop the action, because if he did, the ball would not travel as far as it would if he followed through with the swing. The idea is to hit the ball with control and force, just as a judoka's goal is to throw an opponent with control and force. The velocity of the action continues because of inertia and gravity. As a result, the defender's body is thrown to the mat, and the only thing stopping his body from traveling any farther is its collision with the mat. At this point in the throwing action, simply landing on the opponent is not an effective use of kime. The attacker must maintain as much control as possible of the defender's body to ensure that the defender will land with control and force so that the attacker terminates the throwing action or has the ability to follow through to the mat with a pin or submission technique.

Makikomi: This is the result of an all-out throwing effort where the attacker throws his opponent to the mat and lands on him. This winding or wrapping action is an extension of the kime, or finishing, action of a 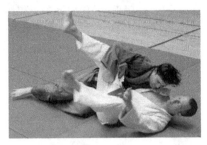 throw. This is a good example of how the attacker and thrower are no longer two separate bodies as they fall but are rather connected together, becoming one object falling through its trajectory until it hits the mat—but with the caveat that one of the bodies maintains control. While it looks to the untrained eye that the thrower is not in control of the action, the reverse is true. The attacker knows where he is going whereas the defender knows where he is going (to the mat) but also knows he's not the one doing the steering. Not every throw ends in a makikomi finish, but it is common in judo, sambo, and any fighting sport that employs throwing techniques. As every judo athlete knows, this makikomi action is common, but it's never an enjoyable experience to be on the receiving end of it.

Differences among Throws, Takedowns, and Transitions

Also bear in mind that the purpose of a **throw** is to put an opponent on the mat forcefully and with control. Force and control are integral goals—and parts—of a throw. The harder a person lands on the mat, the more starch is taken out of him. A hard landing can end a fight immediately (and this is why ippon is scored for a successfully executed throw). This differs from the goal and application of a **takedown**. A takedown's primary purpose is to take the opponent to the mat and then exert further control over him. A takedown can certainly result in a hard landing for the defender, but the takedown's purpose is control, not force. Once the athlete takes his opponent to the mat, he will work to secure a ride (as in wrestling) or other controlling method. This differs from a **transition** where the attacker takes his opponent from a standing position to the mat with a specific purpose in mind. A good example of this is when the attacker uses yoko tomoe nage (side or spinning circle throw) to get his opponent to the mat in order to immediately apply juji gatame (cross-body armlock). Keep in mind that all of this is fluid and dynamic in application. An example of this fluidity is an attacker throwing his opponent with the intention of ending the match in ippon but the defender managing to turn out and land on his front side. The attacker now follows up and transitions from an upright or standing position immediately into a rolling strangle or armlock. This transitioning from standing to the mat is done with as much control as possible on the part of the attacker.

Breakdowns and Applying Technical Skill in Newaza: Next we consider taking an opponent from a stable to unstable position. The best way to think about a **breakdown** is that it is a throwing technique done in groundfighting, and in fact, the principles of kuzushi, tsukuri, kake, and kime are used just as much in ground-fighting as in throwing techniques. When using a breakdown, the attacker takes his opponent from a stable base to an unstable base. This is the same thing that happens in a throwing technique. The term "breakdown" is a generic description of this action. The phrase **hairi kata** (entry form) is the generic name used in judo for this action of controlling movement when entering into a technique. In judo, the word **turnover** is used to describe rolling an opponent over onto his back, and this is an accurate description of what takes place. But, in the way in which it is applied, a turn-over is actually a breakdown. A breakdown can be applied from any starting position or posture and does not always turn an opponent over onto his back. In this sense, hairi kata describes what takes place in a breakdown. This sequence of photos of a standard application of juji gatame shows a breakdown in action—taking an opponent from a stable base to an unstable position.

In the first photo, the attacker is in the newaza starting position.

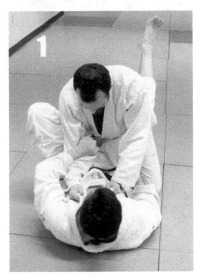

The attacker spins under his opponent and starts to gain more control by using his hands and arms to trap the opponent's arm to his torso and by using his feet and legs to trap and control the opponent's head and body. Look at how the attacker rotates under his opponent. This rotation creates the torque necessary to roll the opponent over and onto his

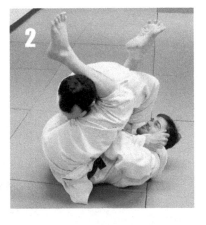

back in the same way that applying kuzushi is used in a throwing technique done from a standing position. At this point, the attacker has also fit his body into position so that the kuzushi phase has transitioned to the tsukuri phase of the sequence.

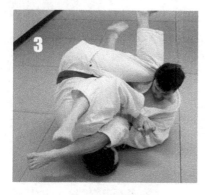

The attacker rotates under his opponent, turning the opponent over and onto his back. The continuation of this breakdown is similar to the kake phase as used in a throwing technique insofar as the attacker is executing the breakdown with control and force.

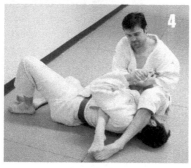

The attacker has successfully broken his opponent down from the opponent's initial stable position to an unstable position on his back. The attacker can now apply juji gatame or another submission technique or pin. This could be considered the kime or finishing phase of the sequence.

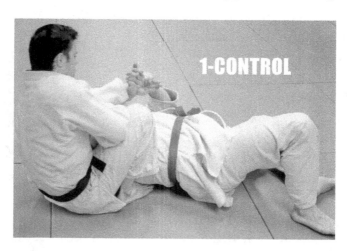

1-CONTROL

Control, Trap, and Apply: Once the attacker has rolled his opponent or broken him down, there are three distinct biomechanical actions used to complete the sequence and secure the armlock, strangle, or pin. These three actions are 1. control the opponent's body, 2. trap the part of his body being attacked, and 3. apply the finishing action (levering the arm free in an armlock, tightening the pressure on the throat in a strangle, or cinching in the arms/hands and securing a base with the lower body in a pin). **Control Phase:** This photo shows that the attacker has broken his opponent down and is now controlling him in this leg-press position. As the attacker improves his position of control, he transitions into the next phase of mechanical skill, which is trapping.

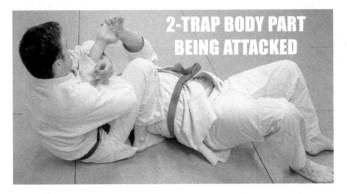

Trapping Phase: As the attacker controls his opponent, his attack is focused on the specific body part or joint that will be cranked, bent, or stretched. In some cases, the attacker may also focus his attack on one of the defender's supporting limbs in an effort to exert more control. In this photo, the attacker uses his hands and arms to trap the defender's right arm to the attacker's torso.

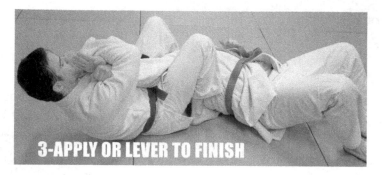

3-APPLY OR LEVER TO FINISH

Application Phase: The attacker secures his trap and transitions into the actual application of the technique. In this photo, the attacker rolls back and levers his opponent's arm out straight to secure juji gatame.

The use of kuzushi, tsukuri, kake, and kime is efficient in both standing situations and in groundfighting situations. They provide a sound foundation and framework, allowing for specific variations based on the context and situation. Now, let's examine the movement patterns used in judo.

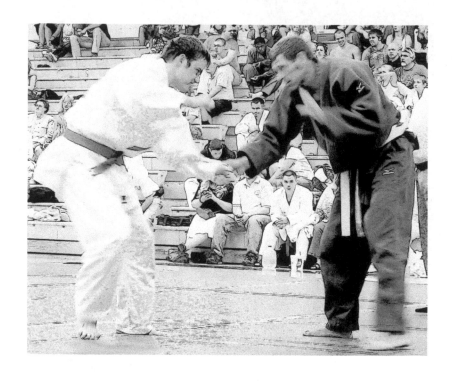

"Small things make big things happen."

—John Wooden

CHAPTER 6

Shintai: Movement in Judo

Shintai: Movement in Judo
Footwork and Movement Patterns in Judo

Jim Bregman, the first US athlete to win medals at the World Judo Championships and Olympic Games once said to me: "The key to effective judo is movement." Jim went on to say that know-

ing how to move and knowing when to move are essential elements of success. Every aspect of judo is based on movement. The more functional and efficient the movement, the better opportunity for success. There are two primary footwork or movement patterns in judo. Sambo and other grappling sports have copied these or made some slight modifications to them. However, these two

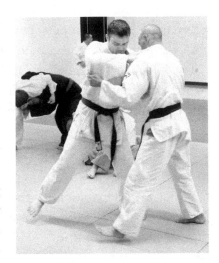

movement patterns were designed by Professor Jigoro Kano early in the development of Kodokan judo.

The first primary movement pattern is **shintai**. The translation implies "advance and retreat," specifically in a linear pattern (either front and back or laterally). A generic translation of shintai is "footwork," as this term refers in a general sense to all footwork used. The second primary movement pattern is **taisabaki**. This is more difficult to translate from Japanese into English but it is roughly "body turning or management/movement." Generically, all footwork in judo is either in a linear direction (shintai) or in a circular direction (taisabaki).

In practical terms, shintai is often used in a generic sense to describe footwork or the movement of the body, so let's concentrate on the following three distinct movement and foot patterns used in judo: ayumi ashi, tsugi ashi, and taisabaki.

Ayumi Ashi: This is a normal step-walking pattern. "Ayumi" simply means "walk." "Ashi" means "foot or leg" and implies the movement of the foot or a pattern. This is a movement where the attacker and defender move either forward or backward in a straight line.

Tsugi Ashi: This is a shuffling or sliding footwork pattern, often at an angle (at the corners) or sideways (laterally) but sometimes can be done in a straight line forward and backward as well. "Tsugi" means "successive" and implies a shuffling movement where one foot meets the other but the feet never cross. "Ashi" means "foot or leg" and implies the movement of the foot or a pattern.

Taisabaki: This is a rotary, turning, or circling movement. "Tai" means "body" and "sabaki" implies "management" or "movement" and suggests preparation for getting into position for a subsequent movement. In this sense, when using taisabaki, the attacker always has an end result in mind—either improving his own position or setting up his opponent for an attack. In judo, the rotational movement of the hips as well as a turning or rotational movement of the body is also part of taisabaki.

The most efficient way of moving your feet about the mat is to use a **suri ashi** (sliding step) type of movement. Be light on your feet, not placing your body weight heavily onto your feet when moving about the mat. As noted earlier, this is known as "heavy feet." Beginners at judo mistakenly place a lot of weight on their feet, thinking that they are planted firmly on the mat. But, in fact they are planted *too* firmly on the mat, which seriously impedes efficient movement.

Using the Feet: Our feet serve as our connection to the mat similar to the way our hands serve to connect us to an opponent. The feet serve as a base used for stability and to initiate force. Even taking a normal step requires force to make one foot follow the other in a normal gait, and this force generation is predicated on having a stable base.

Generation of Force: The action of the attacker's feet (or foot if one foot is the driving foot) pushing off the mat is the cause of force. Force is the action that changes the state of movement—for our purposes, the movement of the human body. In a throwing technique, the attacker initiates his movement by driving off one or both feet in the direction of the attack. One or both feet serve as the primary mover in the generation of force. So as the attacker's feet drive off the mat to generate power, he will also use his feet to direct the movement his body.

Change of Direction: As the attacker pushes or drives off his feet to enter into his throwing attack, he will push into the direction necessary to 1. break his opponent's balance by use of this movement (kuzushi) and 2. continue to move in order to fit his body into position to make the throw happen (tsukuri). Often, the attacker will initiate his body movement in one direction and suddenly change the direction of his body in order to facilitate the next phase of the attack. The feet will move initially in one direction to get the body in motion and then will be used to change the direction of movement and generate force in the new direction.

The combination of generation of force and directional change controls the velocity of the movement—remember that velocity is the combination of speed and direction of the motion—and is dependent on a stable base from which to launch the attack.

Don't Be Flat-Footed: In order to generate force and change the direction of movement, the part of the attacker's foot or feet in contact with the mat is important. It's important not to be flat-footed where the entire foot is in contact with the mat and the weight of the body is bearing directly down. Being flat-footed means the feet are of little use other than to provide stability. Foot movement should be graceful and purposeful. The front of the foot (the ball of the foot and the toes) should be the primary area making contact with the mat most of the time. In order to generate force, the athlete will drive off the ball and toes. Likewise, in directional change, the athlete will rely on the ball pivot when changing direction. It should be added that driving off the ball of the foot and toes is used in the same way in groundfighting. A good way to think about your feet is that they are similar to your hands. Both the hands (with their fingers) and the feet (with their toes) are the appendages extending from either the arms or the legs. The hands grab and control the body of an opponent in a way similar to how the feet grab the mat and control movement.

Stability and Base: The two feet standing and connected to the mat form the base of the human body. Stability is produced by the even distribution of weight on each side of a vertical axis. Stability is also the ability to withstand change when an outside or opposing force (for our purposes, an opponent) attempts to upset the body's equilibrium. **Equilibrium** is the position of the human body in which opposing forces are equal to each other. The base is the foundation or primary support structure of any object and, in our case, of the human body. This is the area formed by the outermost points of contact of the athlete's body with the mat.

The distance between the feet and the distribution of body weight are important for optimal stability and balance. The general measure for optimal distance between the feet is that each foot is in a reasonably direct line extending from the hip to the mat. When moving about the mat, the athlete should attempt to not let his feet get either too close or too far apart from each other. Crossing the feet produces a highly unbalanced condition and the feet get "tripped up" on each other and are useless for efficient or effective movement, stability, and balance. When the feet are positioned optimally, the athlete will be better able to distribute his body weight efficiently. In most situations, the weight placed on each foot is even, but the distribution of body weight on each foot is dynamic as the athlete steps or moves. Each foot will take turns bearing a different portion of the body's weight as the athlete moves. The feet serve as the conduit that connects the athlete to the mat, providing stability, the generation of force, and directional movement. An athlete spending extra time on footwork drills and moving about the mat (both with and without a partner) is time well spent in the development of efficient and optimal technical skill and control of his own movement and the movement of opponents.

Using the Feet in Judo the Way a Boxer Uses a Jab: Bruce Toups, a great coach and former director of development for US Judo, once told me: "Use your feet like a boxer uses his jab." I've heard other coaches say this as well, and it is good advice. What is meant by this is that judo athletes will use foot movement, sweeps, and "probing" to set up a bigger attack. From its early history, Kodokan judo relied on **kowaza** (small or minor techniques) in the form of foot and leg throws as a principal attack or to set an opponent up for the major attack (**owaza**). Using a ko uchi gari (minor inner reap) to elicit a response from an opponent in order to attack with a seoi nage, uchi mata, or tai otoshi is like a boxer using his left jab to set his opponent up for his straight right or left hook. Using these foot movements as an actual attack or as a feint make up **renraku waza** (combination techniques), which we discuss below.

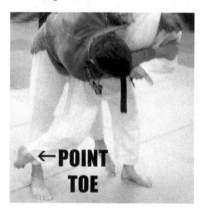

←POINT TOE

Pointing the Toes: This action serves as an effective method of control over an opponent's limb in both throwing attacks and in groundfighting. This movement of pointing the foot down is called **plantar flexion** and serves as both a method of control and generation of power in throwing techniques. The gastrocnemius, soleus, and the other muscles of the lower leg are directly affected when an athlete flexes (points down) his foot so the toes are pointed downward or to the mat. This action causes the muscles in the lower leg to be at their maximum muscle contraction (shortening). This contraction generates additional power into the throwing movement and serves as a useful means of control with the foot and lower leg. In a similar fashion, the attacker using his foot to point and "wrap his foot" around his opponent's ankle when performing foot sweeps allows more control of and power behind the sweeping leg.

Continuity in Movement: This applies to all phases of judo, but a good way to explain it is through considering renraku waza (combination techniques) and renzoku waza (continuation techniques). These are the throwing attacks where two or more throws are linked together. Let's look at the difference between these two types of controlling movements.

In a **renraku waza (combination techniques)**, the attacker launches an initial throwing attack. This attack may be a real attempt to throw his opponent, but the opponent blocks or evades the attack. The attacker then switches to another throw, but in the opposite direction of the initial attack. For instance, the attacker hits in with a ko uchi gari (minor inner reap) and the opponent hops around to evade the throw. The attacker reacts by using a seoi nage (shoulder throw) to throw his opponent. So, in this case, the attacker made a real effort to throw his opponent with ko uchi gari, but the opponent evaded the attack, and the attacker followed up with his second attack, a seoi nage, and threw his opponent in the opposite (or in a different) direction of the initial attack. Another variation of renraku waza is when the attacker fakes or feints the initial throw or movement to elicit a response from this opponent and then follows up with a second attack, often throwing the opponent in a different direction than the initial feint. An identifying feature of a renraku waza is that the initial attack or movement is focused in one direction and the

follow-up technique is a different technique and usually focused in a different direction.

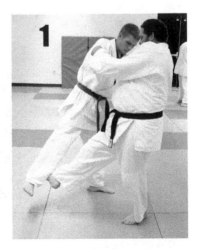

1. The attacker feints with a ko uchi gari as his initial movement. This ko uchi gari attack would throw the defender backward. The attacker uses his ko uchi gari feint to draw the defender's stance wider and possibly even lure the defender to hop around to avoid the leg attack.

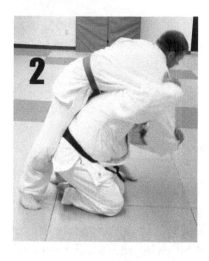

2. As the attacker opens his opponent's stance wider, the attacker attacks again, this time with a seoi nage, reversing the direction of the attack from a rear throw (ko uchi gari) to a forward throw (seoi nage).

In a **renzoku waza (continuation techniques),** the follow-up attack is a continuation of the initial attack. The attacker will either make a real initial attempt to throw his opponent or use a feint to elicit a response. As the defender evades or blocks the initial throwing attack, the attacker will hit in immediately with a second throw as a continuation of the initial attacking movement, often (but not always) in the same direction or movement pattern as the initial attack.

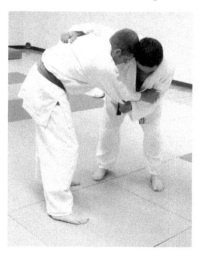

1. A good example of a renzoku waza is the use of **ken ken** (hop hop) in a throwing technique. There are two primary instances where ken ken is used. One is where the attacker's initial attempt at a throw does not materialize, and he repositions his body by using a series of short, choppy steps to continue the attack. The second instance is when the attacker initially feints or fakes an attack to elicit a reaction by the defender and then uses a series of short, choppy steps to continue the attack. In this photo, the attacker (right) attacks his opponent with o soto gari.

2. The opponent resists, or the attacker may have used his attacking foot/leg as a feint. The attacker uses his left foot/leg (the supporting or driver foot/leg) to hop forward using a ken ken hopping action of short, choppy steps for stability in continuing the attack.

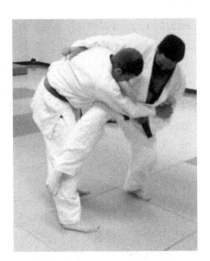

3. The attacker continues the attack without pause and drives his o soto gari in deeper to complete the throw. This continuation, without even a slight pause in the technique (both throwing and in groundfighting), is what defines a renzoku waza.

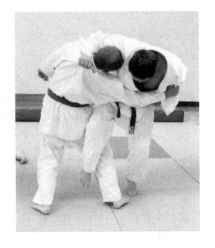

The "Changeup": An effective continuation technique is the "changeup," where the attacker surprises his opponent and fakes an attack from the right side and then immediately switches to the left side to throw him. Much like a baseball pitcher uses a changeup and throws a slider when the batter expects a fastball, a judo athlete can use this tactical approach to renzoku waza. The attacker can also use this changeup tactic in abruptly changing the direction of his initial movement and switching to a different direction to make his attack.

The "Double Take": A renzoku waza, sometimes called a "double take," is when the defender avoids the initial attack, and the attacker immediately attempts the same throw a second time with no pause in the action. An example is when the attacker does a seoi nage and the defender does a hop-around type of avoidance move only to have the attacker hit in again with another seoi nage. The defender's hopping action to avoid the throw gives the attacker room to gain momentum and attack more strongly the second time. This is a simple yet effective technique where the attacker uses the same throw twice in a row without pause.

Control: Control is manipulating or moving an opponent so the attacker dictates where and how the opponent reacts as well as manipulates the consequences of the attacking (throwing) action. In other words, the attacker dictates how, where, and when the defender moves.

Force: Force is the generation of power by the attacker (power results from speed, strength, and acceleration). Force is necessary to move an object (in this case, a human body). A push, pull, or other movement that changes the motion or movement of an opponent's body is force. Overcoming the defender's resting inertia requires force. Force is also the result of the falling action of the human body. It is important enough to say again: the two goals to achieve in every technique—be it a throw, pin, or submission—are control and force. This is why **ippon** is scored for a technique that has achieved both. As Rene Pommerelle said, "You can throw somebody, or you can *throw* somebody."

Every action in judo is movement; some are big and some are small. Every movement has a function, and each movement leads to another movement or is the result of a preceding movement. The athlete who better uses, applies, and controls these movements in combination with one another will be successful. For more analysis on movement, please refer to chapter 9.

For an athlete or student to learn, retain, and master the controlling of movement, he must have a place and opportunity to do it. The place that affords the opportunity is the judo club, and it's the coach at that club who is responsible for imparting the knowledge and seeing to it that the knowledge is retained and refined. Let's now take a look at some aspects of teaching and learning movement.

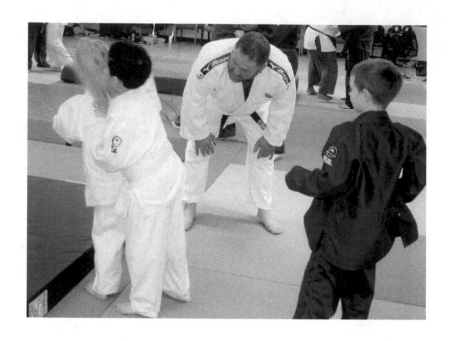

"The first time is cognition. The second time is recognition."
—Marshall McLuhan

CHAPTER 7

Teaching and Learning How to Control Movement

Teaching and Learning How to Control Movement

This book is not only about how to control movement; it is also about how to *teach* movement. So, at this point we will examine some methods that might be helpful in teaching judo movement and discuss some traits that make for effective coaching. A coach doesn't have to be a world champion to develop world champions. However, it is the responsibility of coaches to appreciate, understand, and show how to perform fundamentally efficient technical skills in order for them to adequately teach those skills. A coach must possess a sound understanding of why and how a technical skill works before he can convey these complex skills to another person. In other words, the coach should know what he's talking about before he starts talking.

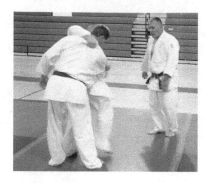

Coaching Is an Art Based on Science: The better that coaches (and students) understand the principles that make the human body work and move, the better they will understand the principles that make judo work. An example is the concepts of kuzushi, tsukuri, and kake that are taught in every judo club in the world. These principles of controlling movement form the basis of the technical application of judo. Good coaching is both science and art. It is a **science** in the sense that everything is based on sound, rational, and empirical reasoning. Good coaching is based on good physical education. And it is **art** in the sense that coaches are working with human beings and, as such, coaches must be creative in how they best teach skills and provide for the needs of their students, athletes, and parents. There is no cut-and-dried formula for working with people. The art is in how you present the science to your students. The photo above shows Bob Corwin, one of the best coaches I know, doing what he does best—teaching judo.

A Word on Coach Education

It should be emphasized that coaching is a serious responsibility and should be done by serious (and mature) people. Judo is composed of many complex motor skills, and injuries can occur. It is the coach's responsibility to ensure that every practice is conducted in as safe a manner as possible. Judo is also a combat sport, so along with the teaching of motor skills and movement, the coach has the responsibility to teach the maturity to know when to use these skills and when not to. This is why coach education is important. There are numerous coach-education programs, ranging from those that treat the subject in a general way to programs specifically aimed at a certain sport or certain audience. To be a coach, it isn't enough to have a black belt; it takes education and experience—and the more, the better.

Patience Is a Virtue

The complexity involved in controlling movement is arguably one of the principal reasons people drop out of judo. Taking repeated and hard falls is another factor, but the difficulty of learning and mastering standing body movement and throwing techniques requires a great deal of patience and effort (as well as qualified coaches who actually teach it well so that it is functional and effective). Learning standing movement and throwing has a long learning curve compared to the short learning curve for groundfighting techniques. A coach's challenge is to retain students long enough so that they are able to perform controlled throwing movements and achieve some success in individual mastery of judo skills (even at a basic level of skill mastery). It takes time, effort, and a lot of patience on the student's part and certainly on the coach's part to achieve this. In today's culture of instant gratification, where quick results are expected, a necessarily slow and sometimes tedious pace in learning how to perform skillful throwing techniques can be difficult to deal with. There are numerous factors that determine success, but one of the most important in learning and mastering the control of movement is patience. A structured and systematic approach to learning skills can help the student to persevere.

Practice: The primary place a person learns judo is at practice. Professor Jigoro Kano said, "Never miss practice." Consistent and regular attendance is probably the most important key to success in judo. If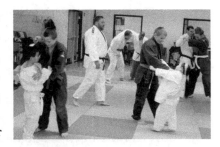

someone isn't at the club working out, he's not doing judo, so he won't get any better at it. It's the coach's responsibility to ensure that practices and workouts are worth coming to. That's not to say the coach should entertain his students. It means the coach should make the practices interesting, enjoyable, and challenging. Not every practice is fun. The coach must recognize the difference between fun and enjoyment. An effective practice will focus on the student or athlete learning, retaining, and mastering technical skill. A good practice will also provide the athletes with a physically challenging workout suitable to age, physical ability, and health. An effective practice must also be appropriate to the students' skill level, maturity, and physical abilities. There is only a limited amount of time that students and athletes are actually on the mat, even if they are elite-level athletes in serious training. Because of this, a coach's management of time is an important factor in getting the most out of every practice. The above photo shows Coach Ken Brink working the mat and moving from one group of students to another to ensure that every student has a beneficial workout. Constant observation by the coach is necessary so everyone has a safe, enjoyable, and productive training experience.

Fundamentals

Without good fundamentals no one can ever go on to more advanced skills. Elite or world-class judo skill is simply the fundamentals performed to their full potential. Teaching fundamentals may not be exciting, but it is vital to the development of the student.

When teaching a skill, the coach must always ensure that the skill is done correctly. A novice student learning a basic throwing technique won't master the skill the first time he does it. It takes time and many repetitions done optimally before it becomes an automatic response. This is where patience is a virtue for the coach. Do not rush the students, but at the same time, don't expect them to have perfect technique immediately. For effective learning of motor skills and the development of muscle memory, the coach should teach a skill, drill on it, and make sure the students perform it with basic competence. It's more important for a student to learn a few techniques with optimal skill than learn a large number of techniques with mediocre or poor skill. It doesn't matter how many techniques a student or athlete "knows"; what matters is how well that student can do what he knows. Eventually, students will learn a variety of basic skills, and with time, effort, and a lot of hard work, they will have gained mastery.

Lesson Planning

The coach should develop an overall plan (called an outline) that includes the overall objectives and goals as well as a timetable for progression of skill. This outline should cover a semester in school or about four to six months in a judo club. The outline should also include all the major skills the coach wants to teach in that time period. From this outline, the coach can develop lesson plans on a monthly or weekly basis. Lesson plans are more detailed about what the coach will teach, what drills will be used, and any specific things the coach wants to include in the practice. Lesson plans can be changed as necessary to meet the needs of the group. It is important that the coach develop lesson plans that progress from one lesson to the next so progression of skill is accomplished.

Sequential Teaching: Teach the Technique by Adding Layers

In coaching, it is both useful and effective to break down the parts of a technical movement so the students learning the skill understand why the parts of the movement are where they are and what they are supposed to do. Technical movements must be presented to the students in such a way that they don't seem too complicated.

Don't take ten steps to perform a movement when five will do—but make sure those five are effective.

There are numerous methods of teaching skill, but the one I will highlight here can be best described as "adding layers" to the movement as students become more familiar with it. This is **sequential teaching**. The technique is taught in a sequence with each part of the movement building on the preceding part and necessary for the part that is next to come. The student progresses from one layer to the next until he achieves mastery of the skill. Here is a description of the different phases of sequential teaching.

1. Briefly describe the skill and introduce it to the students. What it is and why it is worth learning. The coach should tell the name of the skill and what it means. The coach should be enthusiastic and "sell" what he is teaching. The coach should also explain what the skill is in such a way that the students will understand the idea behind it and be eager to learn it.

2. Demonstrate the skill in its entirety. The coach will demonstrate, or have one of the advanced students demonstrate, the skill. Perform it at regular speed first and do it again at a slower speed to allow the students a better look at it. It is important not to try to modify the skill to impress the students. Do the move and do it in a fundamentally correct way.

3. Demonstrate and explain the major parts of the skill. Don't go deep into the details of it yet. Explain each major part of the movement. If there are questions, answer them at this point, but stay with the basic structure of the skill. Don't get too far into the specifics yet.

4. Allow time for the students to learn and practice the skill. The coach (and assistants if there are any) should go around to the different pairs of students and provide coaching and feedback of a general nature. As the students begin to grasp the basic structure and movements of the skill, bring them back for more instruction.

5. Demonstrate and explain the skill in more detail at this point. The coach will go into more specific instruction if the group of students is ready for it. If the students still need more work in the very basic and gross motor skills of the movement, go back to working on that. After this more detailed instructional time, pair the students up once more and let them start practicing it again.

6. Allow more time for the students to work on the skill, this time with more specific instructions from the coach on how and why the movement should be performed as it has been taught.

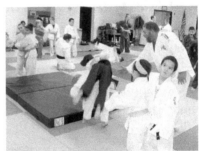

Once the basic structure of the movement has been introduced and the student has practiced it, the next step in learning the movement is to make it functional.

Mastery of the Basic Structure or Form of the Technique

This takes time, patience, a lot of drill training, and loads of practice! The student goes from rudimentary ability to better skill against a nonresisting partner and on to improved skill with a resisting partner (usually in randori). As the student progresses in these levels of skill mastery and has confidence in the movement as well as in the ability to use the movement in randori, he gains mastery of the basic structure and form of the movement. Don't mistake what is said here. The student is not a "master" of judo. He has simply achieved mastery of the basic way of doing the technique. The next phase in learning is to make the technique work for the student.

Adapt the technique so it is functional for the student performing it. At this point, more individualized attention is necessary for the coach to identify how to modify the movements of the basic form of the technique to make it more effective for the individual student. Is the student tall and lanky? Is the student short and squat? Is the student physically strong—or weak? This is when the coach also allows the student a wider range of options for how to perform the movements of the technique. Some students will (without knowing or thinking about it) automatically adapt the technique so it works best for them. If the coach sees this happening and judges that it is biomechanically sound, the coach should encourage the student to make such modifications.

Refine the technique so the student develops his own style of doing it and thereby attains optimal functional skill in the movement. After identifying how the technique should be adapted to be optimally performed by the student, the coach and athlete should spend time in refining the move—just small things here and there—in an effort to make the technique fit the athlete like a glove. This level of skill is what is known as **style**. The athlete has his own style of performing the technique so that it works against resisting opponents with a high rate of success. Essentially, the learning and refining of technical skills will never stop as long as the athlete continues his interest in judo. As he changes physically, he will continually make minor alterations to the skill to ensure that it remains functional and useful for him. This is what Maurice Allan meant when he said, "Make the technique work for you."

So, progressing from the basic application of a technique, we have added layers to it, making it a functional skill with practical application.

Drill Training to Teach Movement Control

Learning and mastering movement and controlling the movement of others are best achieved by the effective use of drill training. **Drill training** is a systematic and progressive use of movements and actions designed to teach and reinforce skill, fitness, and tactical ability. A drill is a systematic method of teaching using repeated movements and the repetitions of specific actions. Through drill training, athletes will learn and retain skills more effectively, and the coach can regulate training time more efficiently. Efficient use of drill training prevents the workouts from becoming stale or boring since different drills provide a variety of situations in training. To a great extent, drill training eliminates goofing off or discipline problems. Drill training provides for a structured practice. A structured practice is essential for effective teaching and learning. If a group of athletes is kept busy, they have less time and opportunity to slack off or play around. In fitness training, an effective use of drills provides a structure and systematic progression of aerobic and nonaerobic conditioning. Drills can be used for tactical awareness and training as well. There are as many different drills as there are situations in judo. A drill can be devised and used for each and every action, situation, or position that takes place in a judo match. A coach can focus on a specific action or situation and invent a drill for it. Drills can also be invented for a group of athletes based on situations or actions that take place or are common in judo matches. An example is for a coach to use different types of drills to teach and reinforce skill in grip fighting. Grip fighting takes place in every judo match. A coach can use a drill that focuses on a specific aspect of gripping or one that permits the athletes to work on more general aspects of grip fighting. The methodology of drill training is based on repetition and development of an automatic response, so let's examine these two concepts.

Muscle Memory: A key benefit of drill training is muscle memory. To be successful, a judo athlete must have an **automatic response**, which is an ability to "do the right thing at the right time." Automatic response takes place when the athlete's muscles have been taught how to perform a specific movement or skill without thinking about it first. For the human body to achieve automatic response, **muscle memory** must be developed. Muscle memory is the same as motor learning, which involves completing a specific skill or task and then neurologically turning it into memory through repetition. The more often an athlete performs a skill in an optimal way, the less time it takes for the brain to process how to do it and, therefore, it becomes more automatic. The key, then, to muscle memory is repetition.

Repetition: This has been briefly discussed earlier in the book but is worth looking at again in the context of muscle memory. A repetition is doing something more than once. Repetition, for our purposes in the context of drill training and skill learning, is a movement pattern performed in a specific way many times. By doing something repeatedly, it becomes a **habit**. A habit is an acquired behavior pattern regularly followed that has become an involuntary behavior or automatic response. A habit can be good or it can be bad. For our purposes, we want an athlete to develop good habits when it comes to how to perform a skilled movement or task. The athlete's behavior must be altered so that he gets in the habit of doing the right thing at the right time. Habit is the same as permanence. Practicing a movement thousands of times creates permanence—a habit. The goal for a coach is to make sure that the permanent habit that is created is one that is most efficient and effective for the athlete doing it.

Types of Drill Training

The American judo pioneer Mel Bruno once told me, "Teach them judo, but train them like wrestlers." In our conversation, Mel advocated using a structured, physically demanding training session emphasizing drill training and structured randori or free practice (in the same way a wrestling coach would train his athletes). The big difference would be to center it all on technically sound judo skill. He also stressed that (paraphrasing) "too much time on the mat is wasted" in judo workouts and that judo students (like any other group of students) need direction from their instructors.

In an effective practice or workout, one training drill leads to another, each adding another layer of development, and all with an overarching or central purpose for that particular workout. Any organized and structured exercise or series of exercises used during a practice is a drill. Every workout should have a goal or objective and every minute spent on the mat should be spent working to achieve that goal. Drill training is the most efficient way of achieving goals in the most efficient use of time.

There are two primary types of drills. The first is a **closed-ended drill** and the second is an **open-ended drill**. There are also subsets of these two primary drills that we will examine.

A closed-ended drill is used to teach or reinforce specific movement or behavior. This type of drill is also called a fixed drill and teaches or reinforces specific behavior within a controlled environment. The athlete repeatedly performs the skill or movement so that it becomes an automatic response in specific situations. This is a more structured drill in terms of permitting freedom of choice in movement. In other words, the coach limits the choices of what the athlete can do in a closed-ended drill; he can only do the specific task the coach has assigned. Both partners in a closed-ended drill know exactly what they have to do and what each partner will do.

In an open-ended drill, the student or athlete has more freedom of choice in how he will react to in an assigned task. **Randori** is an example of an open-ended drill. Randori is "free practice," and while the name implies freedom of choice in movement, it is very much a drill. Randori must always be supervised and have a purpose in the same way as any other drill. Randori in judo is the same as a scrimmage in football or a sparring session for a boxer.

There are other commonly used subsets of these two primary types of drill training.

Skill drills are what the name implies: exercises where the primary goal is to teach and reinforce skills. These drills are not confined to teaching or reinforcing judo techniques. For example, teaching a child how to perform a cartwheel or other tumbling type movement is included in a skill drill. A common example of a skill drill that is done in all judo clubs is practicing ukemi. There is a structure to the act of lining up and taking turns doing rolling breakfalls down the mat. This structure and the regularity of the exercise fulfill the criteria for being a drill.

Situational drills are used to teach and reinforce both technical and tactical skills. This is also called a **variable drill**. In one type of situational drill, the coach will develop a drill based on an actual situation that takes place in a match. As a lead-up to this drill, the athlete has already been instructed on the best response to the situation. A common example is that during a randori period, the coach will give one athlete a higher score than his partner. The coach will instruct the athlete who is leading to keep his lead and instruct the athlete who is behind in the score to catch up and take the lead in the score. A second type of situational drill is when the coach purposely puts the athlete in a difficult situation and it is up to the athlete to elicit the optimal response to the situation. An example is for the coach to have a training partner control the other athlete (who is the focus of the drill) in a strong ride in groundfighting. The training partner's job is to provide varying degrees of resistance according to the coach's instructions. The athlete who is the focus of the drill must have an effective response to get out of the bad situation and turn it into a good situation for himself. Prior to doing this situational drill, the coach has instructed the athlete how to perform the skills that are now being drilled on.

Fitness drills are any drills or exercises that are not primarily skill based but are used to improve flexibility, strength, cardiovascular capacity, speed, agility, or coordination. Fitness 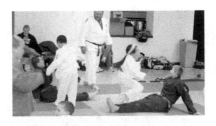 drills are also the warm-up exercises (**junbi-undo**) and cooldown exercises (**shumastsu-undo**) that are performed at every practice. These include flexibility exercises and any mat games. Mat games are useful tools for a coach, as they allow the students to "let off some steam" and have fun. As a coach, I use mat games at the end of our workouts as both a reward for the students' hard work and as a useful skill in fitness training (on a more occasional basis) as a warm-up at the start of a practice. Mat games are enjoyable and beneficial for both children and adults.

In every drill, value carries over from one type of drill to the other. For example, skill drills involving rolling breakfalls or cartwheels can also serve as fitness drills.

As we've observed more than once in this book, teaching is an art based on rational science. To make the mechanical movements of judo work, the person doing them must apply them so all the individual pieces of the movement fit together like a puzzle. One of these pieces is presented next, the tsurikomi action.

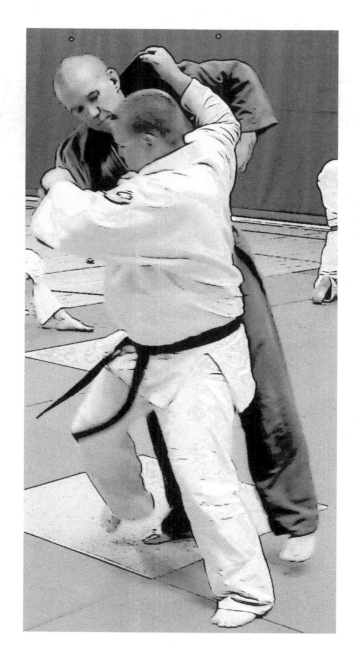

"*There are no good tricks in judo, only good techniques.*"
—Bob Corwin

CHAPTER 8

The Tsurikomi Action

The Tsurikomi Action

A key part of every throwing technique is how the attacker uses his hands and arms in connection with his hip movement, the turning action of his body, and the use of his leg or foot movement. This action is the primary method of "setting up" an opponent for a throwing technique and is called tsurikomi. Tsurikomi is the lifting-pulling action that is essential in transferring force from the attacker to the defender.

Importance of Gripping in Exerting Force and Control: Transference of Force from Attacker to Defender

The first thing we touch an opponent with is our hands; this is why the use of the hands, arms, elbows, and shoulders, as well as the use of movement, are essential in exerting force and control over an opponent. The

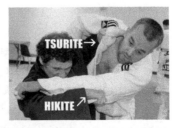

hands and arms are one (but not the only) method of generating as well as transferring force from the attacker to the defender. This means it is incumbent on the athlete and coach to train in both power and skill work in order to maximize the transference of force. The role of the hands and arms in gripping, grabbing, and manipulating an opponent is of vital importance. Each hand and arm works separately yet interdependently to achieve maximum control over the opponent.

Using the Hands for Control: Remembering that the hands are the part of the attacker's body that most often makes first contact with the opponent and, as a result, the primary task of the hands is to control, the attacker will make any number of movements and adjustments in hand position to exert and maintain control. In many situations, the attacker will use his hands to jerk or snap the opponent. An example is that the lifting-pulling action is done with a "snapping" or "jerking" movement initially, and this quickly transitions to a more precise pulling action with his hands, steering the defender in the direction of the throwing movement. This initial jerk takes the defender off guard long enough for the attacker to establish his primary pulling or pushing movement.

In judo, each hand has a specific use and name that describes that use. The **hikite** is the pulling hand (also commonly called the sleeve hand). Hiki translates to "pull" and te translates to "hand." The hikite does a lot more than simply pull, and we will examine its use more fully. The tsurite is the lifting hand. **Tsuri** means "to lift" or "to suspend" as in holding and controlling something to lift or hang in the air. The tsurite has more uses than only lifting, as it also steers and manipulates an opponent. It is commonly called the "power hand" or "steering hand" because it does indeed transfer power from the attacker's arms and body to the action of the throw. It also steers or guides the defender into the direction of the throw. World Judo Champion Neil Adams refers to the tsurite as the direction hand and the hikite as the control hand, which are excellent descriptions of their actions.

Tsurikomi Entry to Throwing Techniques: The action of tsurikomi is not limited to the use of the hands, arms, and upper body. The entire body and movement of the attacker is part of effective tsurikomi. The lifting and pulling action of hikite and tsurite suspends and controls the defender's body long enough to allow for a coordinated hip-turning movement (taisabaki) and simultaneous move-

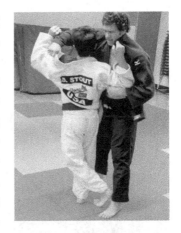

ment of the feet. This entire combined movement is what is known as "tsurikomi" and is the most fundamental method of entering a throwing technique. There are other effective gripping, movement, and footwork patterns for throwing techniques, but this is the movement pattern most students and athletes learn, practice, and use. It is such a fundamental entry method that it can be said that the second phase of a throwing technique (tsukuri) is not possible without the effective application of tsurikomi. In this photo, look at how the attacker uses a coordinated and total-body approach to the tsurikomi action. The attacker's hips are in optimal position to complete the turn because of the attacker's effective use of his hands and arms, along with his foot movement. Since the hips are attached to the legs and feet, the attacker will use rotary power to turn and execute the throw.

The rotation or turning of the attacker's hips is one of the primary drivers of torque in a forward-throwing technique, but this hip turning (taisabaki) action is greatly assisted by the attacker's use of his feet. The classic tsurikomi entry's use of an immediate and explosive back step is called **fumikomi** (stepping

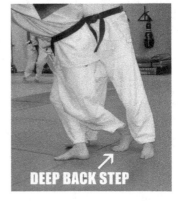

DEEP BACK STEP

or stomping in placing most of the weight into the stepping foot). This fumikomi action must be a fast, explosive movement. Used in many throwing techniques, it serves several key functions:

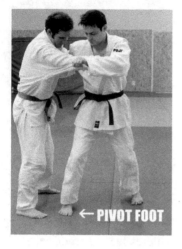
← PIVOT FOOT

1. It permits the attacker to more fully rotate or turn his hips into the action of the throw, thus providing torque.

2. As the attacker steps back with his foot, he does so with a forceful action—a stomping action onto the mat. This stomp puts power into the movement that is transferred through the attacker's leg into his hips and upper body.

3. It permits the attacker to close the space between his body and the defender's body, especially at the hip area near the defender's center of gravity. This deep back step is done in conjunction with the attacker's use of his hands in the lifting and pulling action (tsurikomi) to control and break the defender's balance and control his movement.

The action and placement of the attacker's lead foot (in right-sided throws, the attacker's right foot) is of prime importance. The attacker does not "step into" the defender but moves his lead foot to "get it out of the way" so he can better move his back foot in place and get the deep back step necessary to enable a strong rotation of his body. In looking at the foot placement of the attacker's right (or lead) foot in the photos, notice how he moved it across his body and not directly forward. One of the major reasons students are not able to get a deep back step and full rotation of their hips in using the tsurikomi entry is that they step directly toward their opponent and their lead foot is placed in the middle of the defender's stance rather than across the attacker's body and in front of the defender's body. The attacker's lead foot now becomes the "pivot foot" because the attacker steps in, placing his weight on the front part of his foot (the ball of the foot) in order to pivot on it, which permits him to start his rotational movement with his hips and move his back foot and leg to step in deeply. At this point, it's also worth mentioning that the attacker lifts and pulls the defender into the attacker's chest. The attacker does not move or step into the defender. This is the tsurikomi movement at work. Look at the position of the attacker's right foot in the photo below. The attacker does not step directly to his opponent but rather steps across his own body and in front of the defender. Look at the body space at the hip area, as the attacker will use the lifting and pulling action to draw his opponent to the attacker, putting the defender's body in motion into the direction of the throwing action. The attacker's lead or pivot foot basically "gets out of the way" so he can move his back leg in deeply and turn his body.

So this combination of the attacker stepping across with his right foot, then pivoting on it as he uses his hands, arms, and rotation of his hips and upper body to lift and pull the defender forward into the attacker's chest area—along with a deep back step and sharp head rotation—all combine to form the tsurikomi 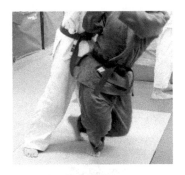 entry. In this photo, the attacker has stepped across and pivoted with his lead foot, allowing enough space to optimally move his back leg in deeply. This permits the attacker to make an explosive rotation of the hips, torso, and head. Notice the forward lean of the defender's body into the direction of the attacker and the direction of the throw as a result of the tsurikomi (lifting-pulling) action.

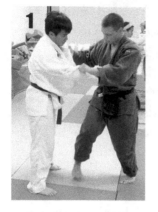

Basic Tsurikomi Entry: This sequence of photos shows an example of the most basic entry form used in judo. There are other entry forms, but this one is the primary skill taught to most judo students. This first photo shows the attacker starting his lifting-pulling action with his hands and arms as he moves his hip, leg, and foot forward. Notice the control the attacker has of his right foot as he points it to his left so that the front of the foot will be placed on the mat so he can pivot on it.

The attacker rotates his hips and torso as he executes a deep back step with his left foot and leg. The attacker uses his hands and arms to lift and pull upward and forward. The attacker turns his head into the direction of the action for added upper-body power and control.

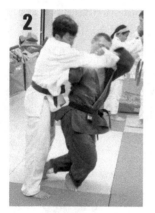

As the attacker rotates into the throw, he lowers the level of his body so he is under his opponent's center of gravity. This "corkscrew" action is an integral part of this entry as it provides additional torque.

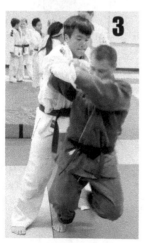

The attacker is now in position to execute the throw. His body position is much like a coil ready to expand and release the kinetic energy that has been generated by his tsurikomi action.

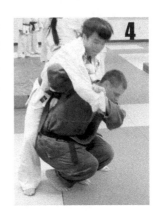

In some throwing techniques such as tai otoshi or a leg-style spinning uchi mata, the attacker will position his back foot and leg outside the defender's stance and body. The attacker still takes a deep back step and uses his lead foot to make the pivot that allows the body rotation, but the deep back step is not placed between the defender's legs but on the outside of them.

This photo sequence shows a basic tsurikomi entry for tai otoshi. In this first photo, the attacker's posture and foot placement (stance) indicate that he is ready to make his attack.

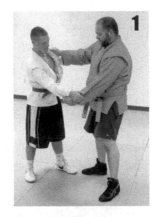

The attacker moves his lead foot across his body—in this case, in the middle of the defender's stance in front of and between his feet. As the attacker pivots on his right foot, he uses the lifting-pulling action with his hands and arms and swings his left foot back and to the outside of the defender's left foot.

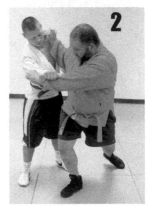

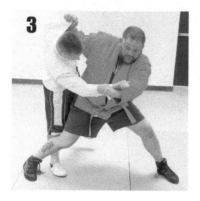

The attacker plants his left foot in a fumikomi action on the mat as the rotational and pulling action of the attacker's tsurikomi movement draws the defender's upper body off balance and forward into the direction of the throw. Simultaneously, the attacker positions his right foot and leg optimally in preparation for the kake (execution) phase of the throwing movement.

Use of the Hands, Arms, Shoulders, and Upper Body in Gripping and Throwing

As discussed earlier in this book, in almost all circumstances the first contact between two opposing athletes comes from gripping and the use of the hands, arms, and even the shoulders. The point of transfer of force and control in most cases is the hands. But gripping or grip fighting is not merely confined to the use of the hands. While the hands are the tools that grab on to an opponent's jacket or body, they are an extension of the entire body and specifically an extension of the arm and shoulder movement of the opposing athlete.

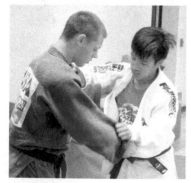

Kumi Kata: These are the forms of grasping or gripping used in judo and any grappling sport using jackets. The name is generically used to describe the gripping action. The common use of gripping the lapel and sleeve is considered the basic method of kumi kata. Prior to Jigoro Kano and Kodokan judo, there was no method in jujutsu for assuming a neutral (or mutually agreeable) grip that provided a starting point for the application of techniques. This "neutral" starting position is now taken for granted as something everyone does in judo but was a major innovation when first introduced.

The Anchor Hand and Attacking Hand: Rarely do athletes grab their opponents with both hands simultaneously. Often they will use one hand to establish initial control. This is the "anchor hand." The anchor hand is used as a temporary method of control to secure or "anchor" an opponent so the attacker can go

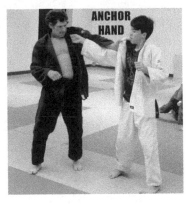

on to gain more control with his other hand, change his posture or stance, or move to gain further control of the situation. The anchor hand may or may not be the hand that makes the initial contact with the opponent, but it is the hand that serves to control the opponent long enough to allow the attacker the opportunity to establish his position and stance. The anchor hand can be used to grip any part of the opponent's jacket or belt. This photo shows how the athlete on the left uses his left hand as the anchor hand to establish initial control. His right hand is the attacking hand. The attacking hand serves to take further control of the opponent's posture and movement. It is generally desirous to get both hands on the opponent in order to control movement more directly, setting the opponent up for an attack.

Using More than Hands in Grip Fighting: The elbows and shoulders are effective tools in blocking, rolling, or manipulating an opponent's hands and arms. In this photo, the athlete

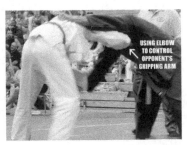

on the left is using his right shoulder and elbow to block and lift his opponent's left arm to negate his back grip.

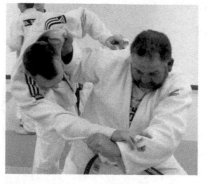

Hikite and Tsurite: We've all heard the old saying, "Get both hands on your opponent!" Conversely, if an athlete is facing an opponent with strong throwing techniques, his coach may tell him, "Don't let him get both hands on you!" In any event, the optimal use of the hands (along with the arms and shoulders) is an integral part of judo. Both hands are important and each has a specific yet interdependent role to play. From a biomechanical point of view, the hands are the extension of force generated by the attacker. This force is transmitted through the attacker's hands into the defender's body. The transmission of power is necessary for the optimal application of a throwing technique.

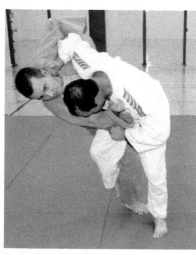

Pulling and Steering: As I have said, each limb—which of course includes both the hands and arms—has a specific yet interdependent role in the application of the skill. For a right-handed athlete, the left hand is the hikite (pulling hand) and the right hand is the tsurite (lifting hand). Mechanically, when controlling the movement of an opponent the hikite does more than pull (although that's its primary job) and the tsurite does more than lift. Each hand, acting both independently and together, steers and controls an opponent's movements in the direction the attacker wants him to go. The use of the attacker's hands often determines the direction in which both the attacker's and defender's bodies will go. In this photo, the attacker uses his hikite (left hand) to make the initial pulling action and immediately uses his tsurite (right hand) to lift and steer his opponent to the angle he has chosen for his attack (in this instance, the defender's right rear corner). Using both hands in this way enables the attacker to rotate his torso and head (beginning with hip rotation) into the angle he has chosen for the attack.

Hikite: The pulling hand (also called the sleeve hand) is fundamentally important in throwing techniques. The elbow of the attacker's hikite is pointed up to allow him more freedom of movement in his rotational and forward pulling action, thus allowing him to 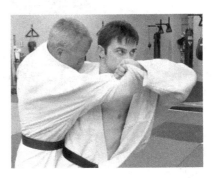 generate more power for the pull. The ideal position for the attacker's hikite hand is when the back of the attacker's hand is turned to his face in the same way he would look at his wristwatch. Doing this creates a strong "corkscrew" rotational effect that puts more force into the pulling action. This hand position also permits the attacker to lift his elbow upward into the forward pulling motion, which also allows for more power in the pulling action. The more velocity the attacker uses in his pulling movement (in other words, the more "snap" he puts on the pull), the more powerful the pulling action will be. This "snap" aids in both the lifting and the pulling action. It does so at the start of the tsurikomi action, where the attacker uses the snap to lock or suspend the defender's arm in place. The snap also aids the lifting and pulling action at the end of the tsurikomi when it controls the direction of movement while adding power to the throw. The hikite's primary purpose is to manipulate the opponent's body so it is projected, lifted, or moved upward and onto the attacker's fulcrum (or axis) and then forward over the axis into the trajectory the attacker has established. While both hands are important in controlling an opponent's body and movement, the hikite is almost always the limb that guides or controls the defender into the direction of the throwing movement.

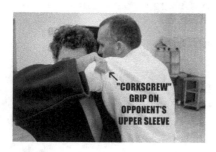

Gripping at the Defender's Triceps: Ideally, the best area to grip with the hikite is the defender's upper arm and triceps area at the back of the sleeve. As the attacker initiates his pulling action, he will rotate his wrist and hand so the back of the hand faces the attacker as if he were looking at his wristwatch. This starts the "snapping" action. Then the rotation of the pulling hand's wrist traps the defender's upper arm and tightens the control of the sleeve. This is the start of the "corkscrew" pulling movement that is essential in generating both control and power with hikite. This photo shows how the attacker grips the upper sleeve of the defender and rolls or turns his hand to tighten his grip on the arm.

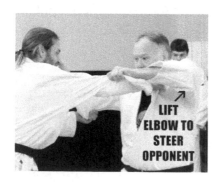

Using the Elbow to Pull and Steer: The attacker's pulling action involves his entire upper body, not only his hand. The rapid rotation of the attacker's torso, generated from turning his hips, is combined with the lifting of his shoulder and rotation of his shoulder girdle area. The attacker lifts his elbow so it is in a straight line with his pulling hand. This positions the attacker's elbow in such a way that it permits an effective transfer of force into the attacker's arm and hand. Pulling and steering with the elbow greatly assist in the pulling and steering action of the hand that is gripping the opponent's sleeve. This illustrates how grip fighting is not simply "hand fighting" but uses the entire body.

Line of Force or Line of Pull: The direction of the movement of the attacker's elbow is critical, as it creates what is called the line of force (or line of direction). The line of force is created by the attacker's rotation of his body 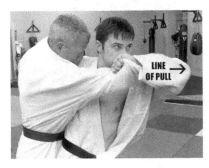 (creating torque) along with direct applied force from the attacker's deltoid muscle in his shoulder. Because of the way the shoulder, arm, and hand are biomechanically constructed, the attacker must always pull with his hand in the same direction that his elbow goes. In pulling, the hand follows the elbow. Conversely, in pushing, the movement of the elbow follows the movement of the hand.

Rotational Use of Hikite: In this use of hikite, the attacker pulls his opponent's elbow and arm into the attacker's body in a rotational downward movement. This traps the defender's arm to the attacker's torso, rendering the arm useless. In this rotational use of the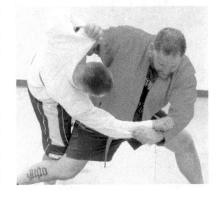

hikite, the attacker essentially pins the defender's arm to his torso. Then, as the attacker rotates or turns into the direction of the throwing action, the control over the defender's arm increases because of the applied force from the shoulders as well as the torque created by the rotation of the attacker's torso in his line of pull.

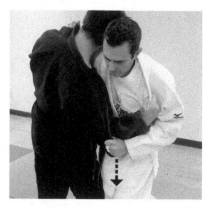

Pulling Down to the Mat with the Hikite: In many throws, the attacker uses his hikite to pull downward to the mat. The attacker's preference may be to pull the defender's elbow directly down to the mat in a straight line or to pull down and into the attacker's torso. The attacker may even steer the defender's elbow by pulling it down and pushing it inward toward the defender's body. In this instance, the line of force is not pulling across the attacker's torso but rather is directed downward to the mat. This method of using the hikite is very useful in throws as different as o soto gari and tai otoshi.

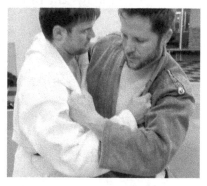

The hikite is not always the hand that holds onto the defender's sleeve. In some throws, the attacker will grip his opponent's jacket (or even belt) at the lapel, shoulder area, or anywhere that provides a stable, strong, and controlling grip. The attacker may pull up and forward, down to the mat, or in a rotational action in the same way he would if he were gripping onto the defender's sleeve.

As the great coach Rene Pommerelle said, "Everything is a handle." This photo shows the attacker pulling down on his opponent's jacket, directly controlling his movement to send him backward in his application of ko soto gake. Any part of the uniform or body can be used to grab and manipulate (depending on what the contest rules permit). Whether by design or opportunity, grabbing any part of the jacket or belt to control the movement of the opponent's body can be useful.

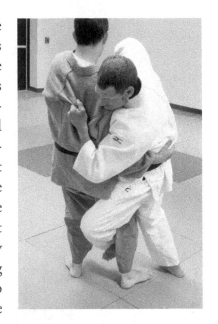

Tsurite: The lifting hand (also called the power hand, the steering hand, or the directional hand) has many uses but its main use is twofold: 1. to lift the opponent's body sufficiently up, forward, backward, or to the side to allow the attacker's body

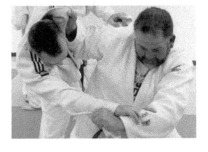

the necessary space to start its rotation or entry into the throw; and 2. to control the trajectory of the opponent's body in the throwing action.

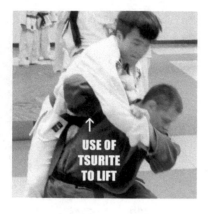

USE OF TSURITE TO LIFT

The tsurite is the hand that not only lifts but traps, hooks, and generally manipulates the defender. In seoi nage, for example, the attacker's tsurite hooks and traps his opponent's upper arm at the shoulder area in addition to lifting it in morote seoi nage (both-hand shoulder throw). The lifting, trapping, and steering action of the tsurite in morote seoi nage shows the multifunctional use of it.

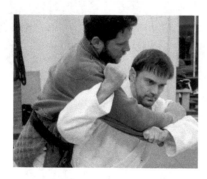

The action of the tsurite is a bit different in ippon seoi nage compared to morote seoi nage. In ippon seoi nage, the right arm—the tsurite—hooks and traps the defender's right upper arm and shoulder but does not aid in the lifting action. This is an example of how the tsurite serves different functions, even in throws that are considered similar to each other.

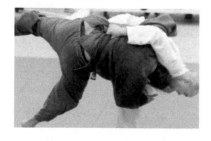

In some cases, especially for tall athletes or when an opponent is bent over or crouched low, the optimal position of the tsurite will not be at the opponent's lapel. This photo shows the attacker using a back grip with the tsurite gripping the opponent's belt. The attacker is using his tsurite to not only lift but to steer his opponent in the direction he wants him to go. Gripping is one of the most important aspects of judo, sambo, or any grappling sport using jackets and belts, so it is wise for athletes to experiment in practice to see which different gripping methods work most optimally in specific situations.

The tsurite is used to trap and control the defender's waist in ogoshi. This use of the tsurite in trapping and controlling is used in other throws as well (such as koshi guruma). The opponent's waist, trunk, and head are useful points of control in hooking, trapping, and controlling in both throwing techniques and groundfighting.

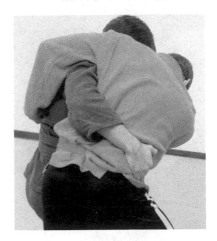

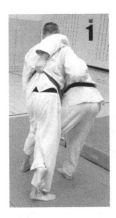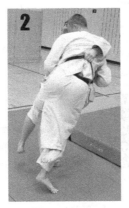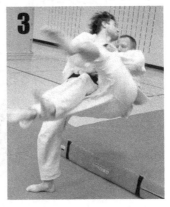

Using the Tsurite in Lifting Throws: In the photo sequence above, the attacker uses his left hand as the tsurite to do exactly what it is named—lift. In this application of obi tori gaeshi, the attacker makes effective use of his tsurite by lifting and steering the defender into the action of the throw. The attacker also uses the tsurite to draw his opponent closer to him as he starts to lift and steer him.

Initially lifting, drawing in, and then pulling, the tsurite steers the defender's body where the attacker wants him to go. Combined with the strong rotational movement of the attacker's torso and head initiated by his hip-turning action, the attacker successfully lifts and throws the defender in the direction the attacker chooses.

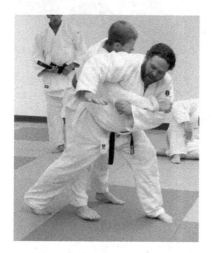

Steering and Aiming with the Tsurite: In some instances, the attacker's use of his tsurite will be primarily to steer his opponent or himself into the direction of the throwing attack. As shown in this photo, when doing throws such as soto makikomi, the attacker does not lift at all with his tsurite but rather uses it like a laser beam to aim in the direction of the throw the attacker has chosen.

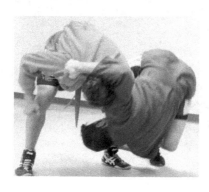

Tsurite and Hikite May Switch: In some throws, the action of the tsurite and hikite may interchange. In the sutemi waza (sacrifice technique) shown in this photo, the tsurite is used to pull as well as steer and direct the defender. The hand that started out as the tsurite ended up being the hikite as the action of the throw progressed. This bilateral exchange of the roles of the hikite and tsurite is not common in most throwing techniques but provides a good example of how fluid a functional application of a throw must be. (By the way, look at the use of the attacker's head in this photo in preparation for what follows.)

Use of the Head: The old saying, "Where the head goes, the body follows" is true and is of fundamental importance in creating both directional control and force in the application of the technique. This is true in throwing techniques and in ground-fighting techniques. In most cases, the rotation of the attacker's head is aligned with the rotation of his hips in the throwing action. Head rotation generates

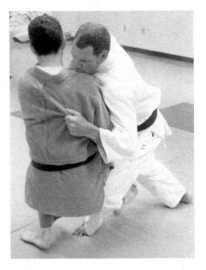

initial force that works in unison with the force generated from the primary movers, such as feet and legs, in a throwing technique. The average human head weighs about seven pounds and this weight provides additional kinetic energy to provide increased power into the actual action of the throw. The head rotation also provides necessary balance in the entire movement, thus giving the attacker the important factor of control in his throwing action. For maximum effectiveness when using the head, the starting posture and alignment of the attacker's body must be optimal. This is why it is important for the attacker to have a straight-aligned spinal structure with a straight back supporting an upright posture. A bent-over posture such as jigotai with a rounded back and head forward of the hips (and center of gravity) is not the ideal starting point for the most efficient use of the head (or any body part in the throwing action). The synchronized power chain that emanates from the feet on the mat, through the hips and torso, and then to the movement of the head is essential for optimal performance of a technical skill such as throwing. This is similar to a shot-putter or discus thrower, where the head is an extension of the body.

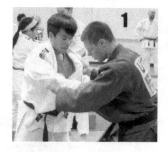

Using the Head for Power and Control: Generating power from the feet, legs, and hips can be greatly enhanced with the use of the head.

1. The rotation of the head in the direction of the throwing movement not only increases the rotational torque produced from the hip and body rotation but also serves as a torque-producing element in upper-body movement. This upper-body production of torque completes the lower body's torque production and creates more power in the technique.

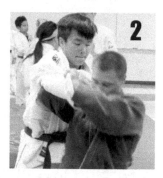

2. As the attacker turns into his throwing attack with his body, his head turns at the same rate of speed. This velocity produced by speed and direction of movement in the upper body of the attacker increases the torque. This creates power in the throwing movement.

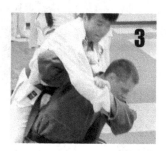

3. The velocity of the head turn also helps in directing where the attacker will throw his opponent. In this sense, the attacker "aims" with his head where he wants his opponent to land. This action of turning the head by the attacker produces a strong and accurate throwing technique.

Using the Head as the "Third Arm": My old coach Rene Pommerelle said that the head is the "third arm" in throwing, and this is certainly true from a functional point of view. The head is an appendage of the body, so it makes good sense to use it for applying control and force. In many cases, an athlete will use his head to exert more control and force in the actual application of the throw as an adjunct to his hands and arms.

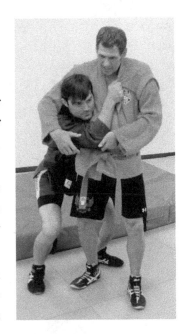

1. The attacker (left) uses his head to wedge in securely at his opponent's pectoral and shoulder area in preparation for using ura nage.

2. This photo shows the attacker using his head as his "third arm" in the application of the throw. The attacker uses his head to form a triangle between his two hands and arms to trap the defender's upper body, giving the attacker more control and opportunity to apply force in the throwing movement.

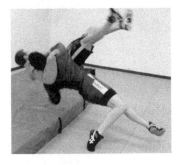

Using the Head to Wedge and Manipulate: This shows how the head can be used as a third arm to wedge in the opponent's shoulder to exert additional control. In some

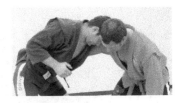

situations, the attacker may use his head to wedge into his opponent's shoulder area to create space or to better use his hands to provide additional control in moving the opponent in the direction the attacker wishes.

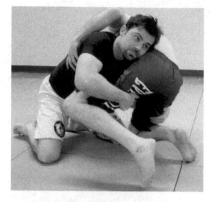

Steering with the Head in Newaza: In groundfighting, the attacker can use his head in the same way as in throwing techniques. In this photo, the attacker uses his head like a third arm to direct or steer his opponent's body in this breakdown.

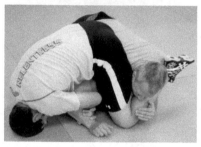

1. What is often called **"posting"** on the head is an effective way for the attacker to provide a stable base for himself in groundfighting. In essence, posting on top of the head creates a wider base area for increased stability. This increased stability affords the attacker more time to control his opponent in order to roll him over into the juji gatame, which the attacker is starting to do in this photo. A key element in the success of this movement is that the attacker is posting on the top of his head, providing for a stable base.

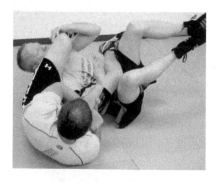

2. This stable base using the top of his head also provides the attacker with a better area of vision so he can change the direction of the roll depending on what he sees and what he feels in the movement of his opponent's body.

3. The attacker completes the juji gatame roll and secures the armlock. Notice that the attacker's head is up and he is looking at his opponent as he applies the armlock. He does 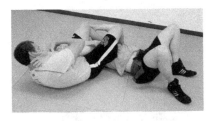 this to have a good look at what he's doing. And with his head up, he can arch with his lower back and hips upward against the defender's outstretched elbow to apply more pressure to the armlock.

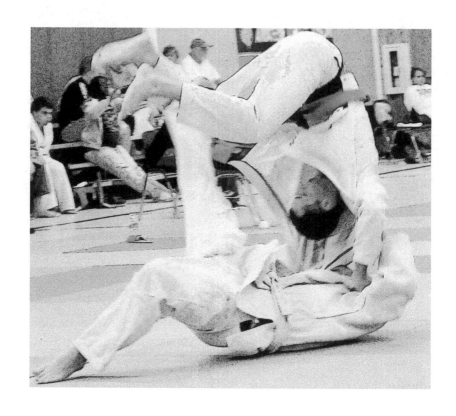

"Your opponent should fear your first attack."

—John Saylor

CHAPTER 9

Movement Is Controlled Motion

Movement Is Controlled Motion

Movement Must Be Functional: Movement is motion with a purpose. Judo is pragmatic. There has to be a reason why you move a certain way or do a certain thing. Not only that, it's important that what you do has a high ratio of success. Every movement must have a purpose and a goal. For an attack to be effective, it has to be done in the most efficient way possible under the circumstances.

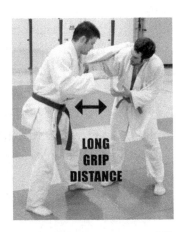

It doesn't always take control to put a body or object in motion. Force alone can do that (such as by using brute strength to throw an opponent to the mat). But it is the controlled force that is generated by the attacker that produces not just motion but controlled movement of both his body and the body of the defender. To be able to use this controlled movement in an optimal manner with a high rate of success takes a lot of training in technically skillful movements.

Linear Motion or Movement: All parts of the body move at the same speed in the same direction at the same time. This is a controlled linear or straight-line movement that occurs in such throws as okuri ashi barai (sliding foot sweep) when using a lateral tsugi ashi footwork pattern.

Angular Motion or Movement: The body parts move at different speeds (the upper body may move faster in a given direction than the lower body, for instance). This is a rotating, turning, twisting, circular, or swinging motion. The human body moves in a circular motion around the body's axis (the axis is the body's center of gravity and balance) much like a wheel moves around its hub or axis.

General Motion or Movement: This is a fairly common movement pattern in judo (or any combat sport for that matter). A good way to think of this is to think of a wagon. The wheels on the wagon turn (angular motion) causing the wagon to move in a specific direction (linear motion). When actually applying this principle, an athlete uses taisabaki (circular body movement) to turn or steer his opponent to make the opponent move in a specific direction. As the attacker turns his opponent in this circular movement, the defender will have to step sideways in a straight line to recover his balance. As the defender makes this step, this is the instant the attacker makes his throwing attack.

Proximity: This is how close the bodies of the attacker and defender are to each other. The space between the attacker and defender is often measured by how far the shoulders and hips are from each other. This is an important concept in judo. How close or how far away an opponent is determines what takes place next. The attacker needs optimal space to launch his attack. He can't be too far away or too close to his opponent. If he's too far away, the opponent will see the attack coming and have both time and opportunity to block or evade the attack and counter with his own attack. If the attacker is too close to his opponent, he won't be able to accelerate sufficiently and develop the power necessary for a successful throw.

If the attacker controls his opponent's shoulders, he will have better control over his opponent's hips as well. This is because the shoulders are situated above the hips, and the structure of the human body only twists and bends so far. In almost every throwing technique, the attacker aims to control his opponent's shoulders. Even when using a sleeve grip, the shoulders are the primary attacking point in terms of control. The arms are attached to the shoulders and the shoulders are attached to the torso, which is attached to the hips. The closer to himself the attacker pulls or manipulates the shoulders of the defender, the better the attacker controls the movement of the defender's body.

When the attacker has direct control over his opponent's shoulders (such as when using a lapel grip or a sleeve grip where the attacker's hands are quite close to the defender's shoulder area), there is minimal space between the bodies of the attacker and the defender. One sees this type of gripping in sambo with regularity where the athletes are often hooked up compactly together, almost appearing to be hugging each other.

A good example of this is what is called "infighting" in boxing when the two boxers are fighting at a very close range with little space between their bodies. This compact infighting is what is called a "short-grip" situation in judo because the distance between the two judo athletes is so short. The distance between the two bodies is often measured at the shoulders. So when two athletes are gripping each other with their shoulders close together, this is a short grip. In many cases, but not all, these short-grip situations result in slower and more deliberate body movement by both athletes. Again, not all short-grip situations produce a slow tempo or pace in movement, but this is more often the case than not.

The opposite of this situation takes place when the space between the bodies of the two athletes is wider. In many situations, one or both athletes will have a low sleeve grip or have their arms extended so there is a wide space between the bodies. This is a "long-grip" situation and often allows more freedom of movement for the athletes. As a result of this freedom of movement, the pace of the match is often faster and less inhibited than in a short-grip situation.

Again, a good way to think about this is to compare it to boxing. When the fighters are really close to each other, banging away with little foot movement, this is infighting in boxing and akin to short grip in judo. When the fighters are doing what Muhammad Ali called "float like a butterfly and sting like a bee" with a lot of space between bodies and a lot of fast foot movement, this is akin to a long grip.

This may seem trivial, but understanding the principle of proximity is essential to better controlling an opponent's movement. Controlling movement in this way is a functional application of situational awareness. Since the bodies of both athletes are constantly moving, it's important for a person to have a trained sense of how to control an opponent in order to get the best technical and tactical advantage. An example of using a long grip or a short grip in a tactical application is when the athlete who is leading in the score may increase the distance between himself and his opponent. He will continue to move about the mat, altering his tempo and looking busy, but the bottom line is that he wants to keep his opponent at a distance, not only to prevent the opponent from launching an attack, but also—and just as important—to kill time and run the clock out. How well he does this and how significant the lead is determines if he can absorb getting a penalty from the referee. This is tactical judo based on the biomechanics of the human body, and it happens all the time. The concepts of short and long grips are not well known to everyone, but they are essential. And these are old concepts used in both judo and sambo. I first heard of short grips and long grips from Rene Pommerelle in the 1970s. These ideas really helped in understanding the use of space between the attacker's and the defender's bodies.

Pace: This concept is also called tempo and describes how fast or slow the attacker and defender move about the mat. In every fight or match, whether in judo or any combat sport, the pace or tempo of movement will speed up or slow down depending on the flow of the action. The rhythm of a judo match is best described as staccato, with its sudden, frequent, and abrupt changes in movement.

Center of Gravity: This is the point at which the mass of the body or weight of an object is balanced in all directions relative to its movement. On the human body, the center of gravity for men is just below the navel and slightly lower for women. Often, the knot of the belt is a good way to determine the center of gravity in judo. When pinning an opponent, the attacker keeps his hips low to the mat to provide a strong 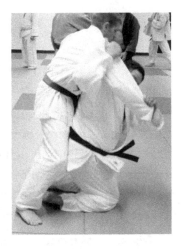 base of support. This also creates more friction that the defender must overcome to prevent any gaps between the attacker's body and the mat that the defender could use to create a wedge with his hands and arms to use to escape. In throwing techniques, the attacker attempts to control his opponent's center of gravity, and in forward throws (especially low seoi nage knee-drop attacks), the attacker must get under the defender's hips deeply to control the center of gravity as shown in this photo.

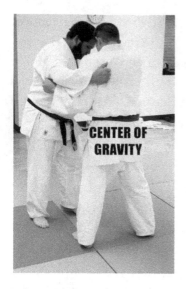

Balance: This is the ability of the athlete to achieve equilibrium with his body in order to maintain control. The defender's center of gravity is relative to the attacker's position and directly influences his center of gravity. A person's center of gravity shifts as the body position changes. Movement causes changes in the body positions of attacker and defender, proximity (how close or far away the attacker's body is in relation to the defender's body), the direction of movement, and speed. As I said before, the center of gravity is at the area of the hips. This is why the movement of the hips is so important for controlled movement in judo. Where the hips go, the body follows, especially when it comes to moving a resisting opponent.

Equilibrium: This describes the action or position of a human body when opposing forces or actions are equal. When this action takes place, balance is achieved. Being able to maintain balance by using enough force to resist the force applied by an opponent is best achieved when an athlete has a strong and stable base. This is true in both standing and groundfighting situations.

Mass: Mass is not the same thing as weight. Weight, when measured on a scale, is a force. This force is relevant to Newton's Second Law that explains how force equals mass times acceleration, due to the pull of gravity. So, the larger the mass, the more space it takes up. Basically, mass refers to how much space an object takes up. Understanding mass is important to better understand how momentum and inertia work.

Momentum: This describes the amount of motion a body has. Momentum takes place anytime an athlete moves. The old saying "the bigger they are, the harder they fall" is true. Momentum is created by the application of force with velocity (speed and direction). Momentum plus muscular force has more power than muscular force alone or motion alone. Momentum creates power. The larger the body (the more mass it has), the faster it will travel in space (through the air) in a specific direction (velocity). The momentum of a falling body in a throwing technique is equal to the mass of the falling athlete times his velocity. The more momentum an attacker has in a throwing attack or roll into juji gatame, the harder it is to stop his attack. The momentum of a body falling onto the mat results, of course, in that body colliding with the mat. This is called **impact**. Impact is what results when two objects collide with each other, such as a human body thrown to the mat. Impact is the ballistic effect or result of force generated and directed into the throwing action.

Inertia: Inertia is resistance to action by a mass or object (for our purposes, a human body). Simply put, if you want to move an object with a large mass (such as a large person), you have to apply more force than you would for a smaller person. This is why heavier people are harder to move than lighter people. There are two types of inertia: resting inertia and moving inertia. A practical definition of inertia is that a human body at rest (in other words, standing still or not moving) has a tendency to not move unless it is acted upon by some external force (for us, this external force is an opponent or another athlete) or does so by itself. Put differently, a human body will stand, kneel, or sit there without moving unless another person forces it to move. Once it's moving (because it's a mass or object and subject to gravity), it will continue to move in a straight line or in the direction it was sent moving. When you start a throwing attack, you want to create enough movement to overcome your opponent's initial resistance—you are turning his resisting inertia into moving inertia and controlling his movement. **This is a description of kuzushi.** Then you continue the attacking movement in order to accelerate (increase the speed and momentum) of your attack so you are better able to form your technique or fit your body into position to throw. **This is a description of tsukuri.** So once you get your opponent moving, keep him moving in the direction you want him to go. This causes both your body (as the attacker) and the defender's body (which are connected together now in the actual throwing movement) to accelerate. This acceleration creates momentum and continues until termination of the throwing action either by a successful throw by the attacker or by a defensive, evasive, or counter movement on the part of the defender. **This is a description of kake.**

To overcome the defender's resting inertia, the attacker must move, force the defender to change his stance, or make the defender change his posture. All of these factors create moving inertia in the defender, which is more favorable for the attacker to launch an effective attack. As discussed in the preceding paragraph, this moving inertia is what is commonly called breaking the balance (kuzushi). If the attacker controls the defender's direction of movement and speed of movement, the attacker will create more favorable conditions for an effective throwing attack. To overcome an opponent's inertia, there are two primary methods in judo. The first method, a direct approach, is **happo no kuzushi**—eight directions of breaking the balance—and the second method is based on the action-reaction method of **hando no kuzushi**, breaking balance by use of diversionary movement (see chapter 3).

Velocity is the description of both speed and direction of the movement in a throwing action. An effective throw accelerates the velocity of an opponent's body (as well as the velocity of the attacker's body who has initiated and controls this velocity). In judo, we must control velocity. Speed is important, but velocity is how fast and in which direction the action is taking place, and it is more relevant to an optimal application of judo technical skill.

This series of photos shows velocity in action in the application of a variation of okuri ashi barai.

1. In this first photo, the bodies of the two athletes are in a fixed place—they are not moving.

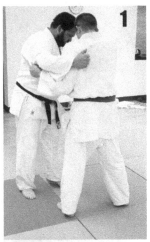

2. The attacker moves to his left (the defender's back is to the camera) laterally and in a straight line with an initial fast speed in an effort to control his opponent's movement so the defender also moves in the same direction.

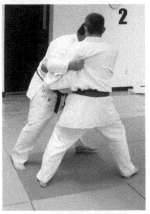

3. The attacker continues his lateral movement and now has control over his opponent. In this photo, the attacker has created the "debana," the right moment, in order to make the attack. This is when the velocity of the movement (the speed and direction) is optimal.

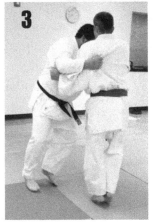

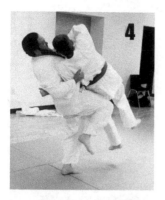

4. The attacker executes his throw. The application of the technical skill must be timed correctly to the velocity of the movement.

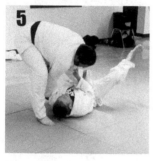

5. The attacker completes his throw, landing the defender flat on his back with force and control, which the attacker achieves by controlling the velocity of the movement.

Speed indicates how fast something moves and **velocity** indicates both how fast and in what direction. While the word "speed" is commonly used to describe the action of a technical skill, it is really "velocity" that is at work. An athlete attacking with a throwing technique wants to not only control the speed of the entire movement, he also wants to control the direction the movement goes in.

As stated before, but worth another look, movement is not just any motion but controlled motion. For our purposes, movement is what we want to achieve, because the attacker attempts to control both the motion of his body and the motion of his opponent's body. This may seem like a small point, but as we have seen, John Wooden said, "Small things make big things happen." Movement is the controlled speed and direction that is produced by the actions of the attacker.

Force: This is any action that changes the state of movement or motion. Force does not always produce movement, but in judo, it often does. The amount of force and the direction in which it is applied produce movement. We'll say more about force later.

Although it's been said elsewhere in this book, it is worth repeating that this controlled motion or movement created through force is called kuzushi ("kuzushi" translates to "break" or "deconstruct" something and implies the "breaking" of an opponent's posture, balance, and stance). This movement creates moving inertia in the defender's body (as well as controlled moving inertia in the attacker's body). Moving inertia is the same thing as kuzushi. The action of the two moving bodies will accelerate or increase in speed and ballistic effect as the moving inertia continues until its culmination. Put another way, kuzushi is the acceleration of movement combined with the direction of movement.

Acceleration: In the popular use of the word, acceleration implies going faster, but for our purposes, acceleration indicates the rate of change in velocity. In other words, how long it takes for an object to speed up (accelerate) or slow down (decelerate) moving in a specific direction. Specifically, acceleration describes how quickly the speed increases and in what direction it moves. Because of the staccato or stop-and-go type of movement we do in judo, as well as the many changes in direction that take place in a match or randori, knowing how to speed up or slow down and change directions is important. For our purposes in judo, we use acceleration in two primary ways. First, in the initiation of a technique, the attacker's body accelerates from a static position and becomes a moving object while the attacker holds on to the opponent and takes him with him. Think of starting an o soto gari attack and driving off the support (driver) leg in an explosive manner. Second, since judo is not done in a straight line (like a 100-meter sprint, for instance), as his direction of movement changes, he will speed up or slow down as necessary to maintain balance and control. This means the tempo or pace of the action taking place in a match is dependent on acceleration. An athlete capable of speeding up and slowing down in his movement, all the while controlling the direction of the movement, is a key element in using kuzushi.

If the attacker controls the defender's velocity (direction of movement and speed of movement), the attacker will more effectively throw the defender. This control of the defender's direction and speed of movement also directly controls the defender's center of gravity. This, in turn, directly controls how close the attacker's and defender's bodies are to each other. It's also important to mention that by initially controlling the grip, the attacker ensures control of his opponent's posture and movement. These three biomechanical factors (grip control, posture control, and space control) are used all the time in judo. Knowing how to use them and when to use them effectively are key to successfully controlling the movement of an opponent.

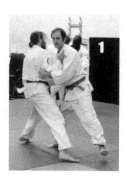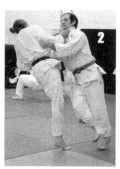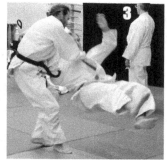

This photo sequence shows how quickly acceleration can occur. Okuri ashi barai is the embodiment of how judo works. The rapid acceleration of force that takes place in just one step creates the power that produces tremendous ballistic effect. Foot

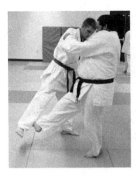 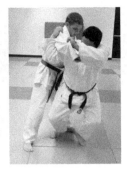 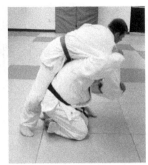

sweeps are based on timing and rhythm, which are dependent upon good control of movement.

Directional Change: As mentioned above, the direction of movement in judo is subject to change in an instant. This is unlike a race in track and field where the action moves in one direction, making it more predictable. Judo doesn't happen in a straight line; any direction is fair game. Velocity must be achieved in one direction and altered depending on the circumstance. Directional change is used often in renraku waza (combination techniques) where the attacker focuses his initial attack in one direction, quickly changes direction, and attacks with another technique. An example of this is shown in the photo sequence where the attacker uses a ko uchi gari (minor inner reap) as a feint to set his opponent up to his opponent's rear side. The attacker immediately switches to a forward-direction throw such as seoi nage.

Another frequently used directional change is when following up as a transition from a throwing technique to groundfighting. A common example is shown in the photo sequence below. The attacker has thrown his opponent, with the action of the throw going forward and down to the mat. The attacker then changes direction to transition quickly to rolling back to apply an armlock like juji gatame or another finishing technique.

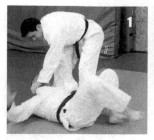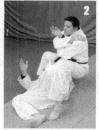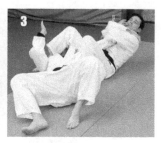

Acceleration and Deceleration in Directional Change: A fundamentally important aspect of directional change is an athlete's ability to accelerate and decelerate as necessary. To achieve a change in direction of the movement, the athlete must decelerate the speed of the action, stop the movement in that initial direction and change the direction of the action, and then accelerate the speed of the action in the new direction. An important element in changing direction is the ability to transfer force when changing from one direction to another. The attacker changes the initial line of direction of force (either pulling or pushing) by using his hands, arms, and torso. This change in the line of direction requires strong and flexible hips to initiate hip and torso rotation and apply the necessary torque that enables the attacker to change directions. This hip and torso strength and flexibility are also used to apply the velocity from that directional change to actual technique used to finish off the opponent. The attacker's feet (including ankle stability) are critical in efficient directional change as the front of the foot and the toes create the surface friction necessary to make the quick and sharp turns required to change the direction of the entire body.

The ability to change direction requires **agility**. Agility, for our purposes in judo, is the ability to accelerate, decelerate (or even stop), change direction, and then accelerate in a different direction—all while maintaining control of your own body and your opponent's body with a minimal reduction in speed. Agility is developed through efficient strength training, coordination drills (on and off the mat), and repeated practice of the skill in the specific movement.

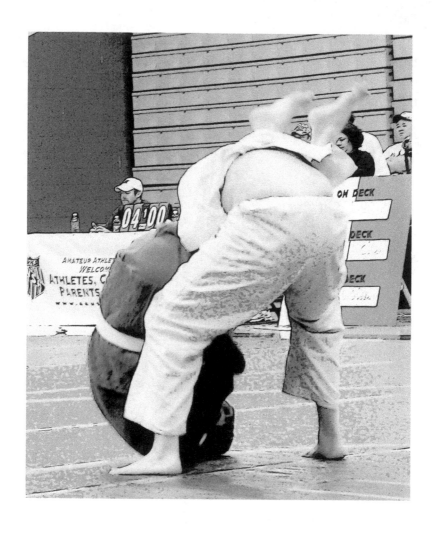

"*Things don't just happen. Things are made to happen.*"

—John F. Kennedy

CHAPTER 10

Using Torque in Judo

Using Torque in Judo

Judo (or any grappling sport) is a contest that boils down to which athlete can apply torque more effectively. The attacker's application of force competes against the defender's resistance to that force. Just like the military uses "force multipliers," we use torque in judo. The better an athlete can multiply his force, the better for him and the worse for his opponent.

Torque: This is the rotation, turning, or twisting movement produced by a force at a distance from the axis or center of a body. Below we will discuss more fully what an axis is. When applying ude garami (as shown in this photo), the elbow of the defender is the axis, fulcrum, or center or the movement. The

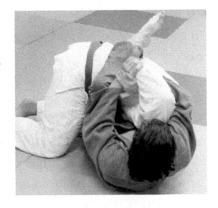

defender's lower arm (acting as a force lever) rotates around the defender's elbow (the fulcrum or axis). The defender's elbow is the axis (or fulcrum), and the attacker blocks or traps the defender's bent upper arm with his elbow/arm that is pressing into the attacker's chest. The attacker uses his hand to apply force and push on the defender's lower arm, creating torque.

Every action causes an equal and opposite reaction. You push and your opponent resists by pulling away; you pull and your opponent pushes. This is important to understand when it comes to moving and turning the human body in relation to throwing it to the mat and is the guiding principle of **hando no kuzushi** (breaking balance by using the opponent's reaction), which we discussed in the last chapter. Pushing and pulling don't always just happen in a straight line; they also happen when turning or rotating.

Rotary Movement: In judo, taisabaki is one aspect of rotary movement and is one of the major movement patterns that govern the technical application of the sport. In practical terms, the attacker wants to move the defender in a circular or turning pattern to get him closer to the attacker's hip and throw him. If the defender resists, this is called **rotary inertia**—in other words, resistance to the turning movement. An experienced judoka will expect this to happen and will use a variety of skills (gripping, controlling proximity or space between attacker and defender, feigning another movement to elicit a response, or any number of things) in order to better achieve his goal of circling the defender in the direction he wishes.

Axis: The axis is the center of an object's rotation. Think of an axis as the hub or center of a wheel. An axis is like a hinge on a door, a fulcrum on a scale, or a hub on a wheel. All action moves around the axis. Imagine looking straight down at someone who is standing below you. Put an imaginary line straight down the person's body from his head to the floor he is standing on. This is the axis or the hub of the human body, and his body rotates around that axis.

Lead with the Hips: In throwing techniques where the attacker throws his opponent in a forward direction (as in seoi nage, ogoshi, and other throws), the rotational movement of the attacker's hip action creates torque. This rotation of the attacker's hips is, as described previously, similar to a wheel, with the center of the attacker's body being the axis. The faster the rotational movement of the attacker's hips, the more torque he generates. Combined with a base of one or both supporting legs and feet attached to the mat and driving from the mat—as well as the turning of the attacker's head into the direction of the throw—this is the primary factor in generating the power necessary for the application of the forward-throwing technique.

1. The attacker's right foot (the pivot foot) is positioned on the mat directly under his right hip. The attacker's primary mover—the first thing he moved—was his right hip in a rotational or turning action. As he did this, the attacker stepped with his right leg and foot, providing a well-balanced initial attacking movement. As the attacker proceeds with his attack, he will continue turning his hips to 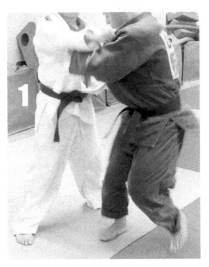 generate torque and close the space between their bodies as he uses his tsurikomi action to pull his opponent to him.

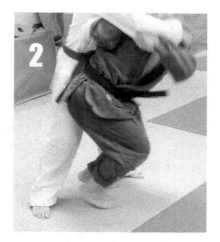

2. The attacker has completed his rotational hip movement along with the tsurikomi action (both in the upper body as well as in his foot movement) to fit or place his body—and his opponent's body—in the optimal position for his seoi nage.

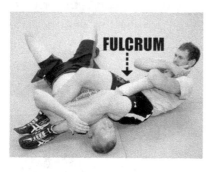

FULCRUM

Torque increases the force applied in acceleration. To make this happen, as the attacker enters his throwing movement leading with his hips, he will rotate the instant his pivot foot makes the pivoting action. If he turns his hips before pivoting, he will lose most of his acceleration in the turning movement, resulting in a loss of torque. The attacking foot—the pivot foot—must also be positioned directly under the hip. (If the attacking foot is the right foot, the right hip is what is being described here.) For optimal effect, the pivot foot does not actually pivot until the hip is positioned directly over it. If the attacker leads with his hips (with the attacking foot or pivot foot directly underneath), he will be less likely to have his attacking foot dangling in front of him only to be used against him by his opponent in a counterattack.

Fulcrum: This is the axis or hinge about which the lever rotates. Think of the defender's elbow when applying juji gatame. The elbow is the fulcrum. When placed against the attacker's pubic bone (which serves as a block), the fulcrum is locked in place (thus, the name "armlock"), and when the lever (the defender's arm) is pulled, the defender experiences pain in the joint and surrounding muscles of the arm.

Lever: This is the name of the barlike object rotating about the fulcrum or axis. Think of the defender's arm when applying juji gatame. The arm is a bar (thus, the name "armbar"). The defender's arm is the lever that is pulled against the fulcrum (the attacker's pubic bone, which serves as a block limiting the lateral movement of the defender's extended arm so only the defender's elbow joint is placed on the fulcrum). Think of this as the defender's upper arm that is attached to his shoulder. When you pull *downward* to apply force against the defender's lower arm and it is blocked against the attacker's pubic bone, the defender's upper arm moves *upward*. This counteraction of force "bars" and straightens the defender's arm. The force arm moves one direction and the resistance arm moves the other direction. When doing juji gatame, keep in mind that the defender's arm is the lever and the defender's elbow joint is the fulcrum. The attacker's pubic bone is actually part of the fulcrum and is called (for our purposes) the block. When the attacker pulls downward or "levers" the defender's arm with the defender's elbow situated on the attacker's pubic bone, the elbow straightens and pain is caused in the elbow joint (as well as in the surrounding muscles and even the shoulder joint).

Torque in Strangles: Torque is used in shime waza (strangling techniques) involving the lapel or other part of the uniform that can be wrapped around the neck and throat. The wrapping action using the

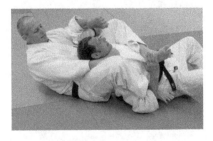

lapel of the jacket is similar to ratcheting a wheel tighter and applying pressure. In this photo, the attacker uses his right hand to apply the torque to the defender's neck and throat as the attacker uses his left hand to control and stabilize the defender's left wrist and arm.

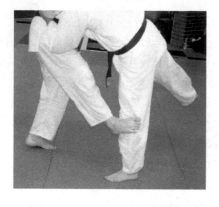

Block: This is the stabilizing object or part of the body that stops, limits, or controls the movement of a lever (for our purposes, a lever would be an arm or leg). An example of a block in a throwing technique is the attacker's foot in a hiza guruma as shown in this photo. The attacker's foot "blocks" or "props" the defender's leg or knee and uses his hip rotation and pulling movement to wheel the defender over the attacker's blocking foot in the application of this throwing technique.

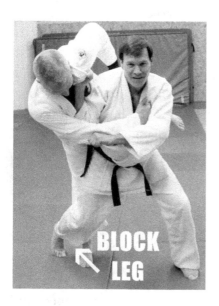

In some forward throws, such as some applications of tai otoshi or seoi otoshi, the attacker uses his lower leg to block the defender's lower leg. In this instance, the attacker uses his lower leg to block his opponent's lower leg in the same way the foot is used in hiza guruma. The difference is in the direction of the throwing movement.

When applying ashi barai (foot sweeps), the attacker's foot is the block that controls the movement of the defender's foot. This shows that the block is not an immovable object but rather a tool that can be directly 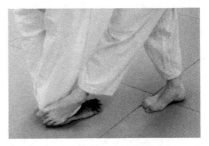 applied to the body part targeted. Also, notice that the attacker's foot is "wrapped around" the defender's ankle for maximum control and not simply used as a club to strike the ankle or lower leg.

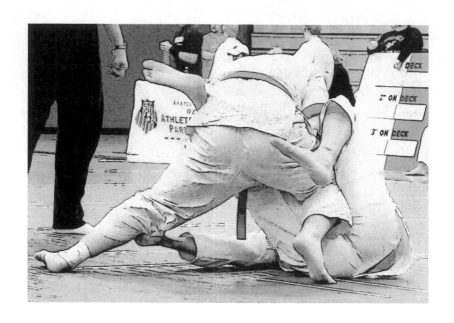

"Flexibility is the key to stability."

—John Wooden

CHAPTER 11

The Human Body's Base

The Human Body's Base

The **base** of the human body is formed by the outermost points that make contact with the mat by any part of the athlete's body, including all appendages (hands, arms, feet, legs, knees, head, or anything else). This is true for throwing techniques when standing and in groundfighting situations. A base works because it is stable, providing a firm foundation for the body. To maintain stability, the athlete must constantly shift his body weight and adjust his center of gravity depending on the circumstances. Let's examine some more factors relevant to base.

Friction: This is the force created when one surface opposes the other. When two objects slide against each other, friction is produced. It is relevant to what we do because this friction provides a stable yet fluid and moveable base for pins such as the

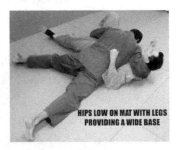

HIPS LOW ON MAT WITH LEGS
PROVIDING A WIDE BASE

one pictured. When holding an opponent in osaekomi waza, the attacker continually shifts his body in order to maintain control for the extended period of time required in judo. This shifting of the body is done to maintain a solid center of gravity required for stability. Friction is also necessary for the attacker to enhance his base by driving his feet off the mat to provide power in the holding movement. The attacker keeps his hips low to the mat for additional friction in holding his opponent. Keeping the hips low also prevents any gaps between the attacker's hips, legs, and torso and the mat.

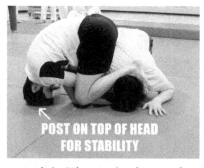

POST ON TOP OF HEAD
FOR STABILITY

Base of Support: The more balanced the base of support, the greater his stability. Usually, the base of support refers to the area on the mat where the feet are (which are positioned directly under a person's body when he is standing upright). This isn't always the case, however. Any body part (or anything) that provides support to maintain balance or to resist the force of an opponent can be a base of support or simply called a base. An example is to "post" or place the top of your head on the mat as you move your body into position to work a head-roll juji gatame or similar move. In this photo, the attacker's head serves as a point of contact on the mat. The attacker positions his body on the defender, who serves as part of the base. The defender's knees and left arm become other points of contact with the mat. The attacker's head and the defender's knees and elbow are the outer edges of the base, providing stability for the time being. The attacker's center of gravity at this point is in the center of his torso between his hips, creating a strong controlling position for him. As the attacker continues his attack, he will shift his center of gravity as he rolls his opponent over.

The base must be stable but fluid and adjust as necessary to maintain stability and control. An example of a base that is both stable and fluid is the one used in holding or pinning an opponent. The hips, legs, and body movement of the pinner must shift and adjust as necessary to maintain a good center of gravity for stability and control of the opponent. Additionally, for our purposes, the base can generate power and is also used as a power base. An example of a power base is that while holding or pinning an opponent, the pinner will "drive" with his feet into the mat to stabilize the body better and hold the opponent down to the mat more effectively. This driving action with the legs and feet is called a **driver leg** or **driver foot**. A driver leg or driver foot is used in both throwing techniques and groundfighting situations to provide power and control for the attacker. In this photo, the attacker uses his left foot and leg to drive off the mat, providing the muscle force necessary to maintain a stable base while he uses his right foot and leg to act as a "rudder" to steer and control the direction of movement used in maintaining this fluid, ever-moving base. The attacker's right leg and foot lying on the mat also serve to add more friction, thus providing a more stable base for the pin. This combination of forces provides both power and fluid stability for successfully immobilizing his opponent for the time required.

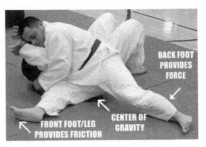

Using the Body as a Base: When fighting from the bottom in newaza, an athlete will often lie flat on his back to provide a stable base for himself. This is used in defensive

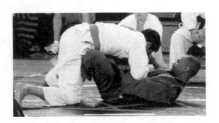

applications of newaza. In the photo, the bottom athlete has extended the space between his body (at the hips) and his opponent's body by use of his legs, feet, hands, and arms. The bottom athlete created this space as a defensive measure and to control his opponent's movement with the goal of adjusting to a different position. Creating this distance between his body and his opponent's body buys the bottom athlete some time to make a better tactical evaluation for his next move. The bottom athlete's torso from his hips to his shoulders is in contact with the mat, creating the friction necessary to create a stable base. Both the bottom athlete's hips and shoulders provide the outermost points of a base on the mat, with his center of gravity in the middle of his back between his hips. Often when fighting from the bottom in newaza, the athlete will make every effort to be round so he is positioned on his hips or buttocks. This permits him more mobility and allows for more aggressive attacks. However, when using this position defensively, the athlete will lie on his back as shown in this photo. This tactic worked for this athlete as he adjusted his position effectively.

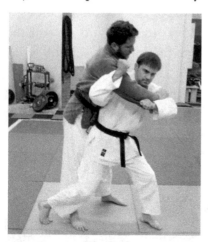

Base of Support Standing: Every position or posture in judo, whether in groundfighting or in standing situations, requires a stable and solid base. Just like in groundfighting, the base must be stable, yet fluid enough to adjust to the frequently changing positions, postures, and situations that take place in a judo match. This power base is used in throwing techniques where the attacker drives off one or both feet to gain velocity and power into the throwing action. When this is done, it is called a driver leg. A base is any body part that supports an athlete's body weight, permits the generation of force, allows the athlete freedom of movement, and, most importantly, provides stability.

Driver Leg and Attacking Leg Depend on a Stable Base: An integral part of the base of support in throwing techniques is the action of each of the attacker's legs. In most throws, the attacker transfers power into the throwing action by use of his driver leg or foot. This is also called the support leg. The attacker uses his other foot and leg to control and manipulate the opponent's legs, feet, or body, and this is called the

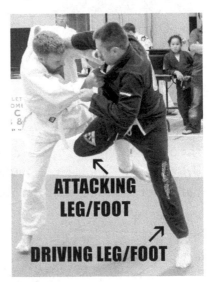

attacking leg. The driver leg not only provides a stable base; it is used as a primary mover that generates power into the attacking movement. This is why it is called a "driver" leg—the attacker drives off it to initiate and continue his attack through to completion. The attacker's foot (the foot of his driver leg) presses or drives against the mat. It drives downward and back against the mat. The force of this driving foot acts against the mat. However, as the attacker moves, gravity works, and as a result a force must act on the attacker's driving foot. This answers why the attacker's body moves into the direction of the throw. The attacker moves because the force of the attacker's foot against the mat creates a reaction force. This explosive reaction force makes the attacker move, driving him in the direction he wants to go. To put it simply, the driver leg/foot works because of gravity and the attacking leg/foot works because it manipulates the part of the body that is being attacked.

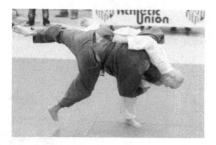

Role of the Support Leg: In this photo, the attacker's left leg has done its work as the driving leg and now controls the movement further by switching its role to that of a support leg. The support leg plays a dynamic role in the throwing action, initially providing the base (think of a pillar in a building) for the attacker to use as a driver and then switches back to being used as a support after the driving action has been accomplished. This action of "support-driver-support" provides a foundation, then power, and then foundation for the attacker's throwing action.

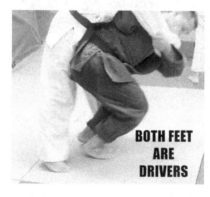

BOTH FEET ARE DRIVERS

Using Both Legs as Drivers—Two Applications: In some throws, the attacker's base is positioned in such a way that power is initially generated off both feet into the throwing action. For instance, this is often the case in low, squatting-style seoi nage attacks or other similar forward throws. The attacker drives off both of his legs like a big spring, creating a ballistic effect and a hard landing for his opponent. Keep in mind that in many cases, one foot/leg will serve as the driver leg. This takes place in throws such as uchi mata, o soto gari, ko uchi gari, harai goshi, and others where the attacker uses his support or base leg as the driver leg to generate power for the action of the throw. You can see examples of using one leg as the driver in other photos in this book. But as shown in this photo, the attacker will drive off both feet and spring into the action of the throw with both legs in the same way a coil unleashes all its tension, creating a ballistic springing movement.

However, in some cases where the attacker starts his attack using both legs to drive off as the throwing action continues, the rotation of the body also continues and one foot or leg finishes the movement as the driver. As an example, the attacker uses a left-sided seoi nage. When both of his feet and legs generate the initial power, and as the attacker's body rotates into the throwing action, the attacker's right foot and leg will become the driver leg.

The Base in Using Torque to Generate Power in Knee-Drop Throws: In knee-drop throwing attacks, the attacker's base is primarily his knees. It is difficult to generate as much power driving off the knees as it is driving off one or both feet. However, if the attacker also uses his feet to generate power, the attack will be more successful. In doing knee-drop attacks, controlling both torque and inertia is vitally important for success. 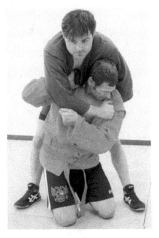 The attacker's initial generation of power comes from the velocity and torque he creates by rotating and corkscrewing under his opponent. A key component in this corkscrew action is that the attacker's toes must be positioned so he is able to use them to drive off the mat, generating power into the forward-throwing action. The attacker wants to spin under his opponent and then drive off his feet to throw his opponent over the attacker's body. As the attacker continues his tsukuri action to fit or place his body into position so that he is on both of his knees and under his opponent's center of gravity, the attacker immediately transfers his power from the rotation of his body to both of his feet, which are dug into the mat. This transfer of power and energy from the attacker's body rotation into his feet enables the attacker to drive forcefully forward into the forward direction of the throw. This spinning-under and driving-forward action produces a great deal of power as well as a great deal of control for the attacker. The attacker must not "flop and drop," allowing the top of his feet to touch the mat. Since the attacker is positioned on both of his knees, he must instead "corkscrew" himself under and below his opponent's center of gravity. If the attacker were to simply drop straight down (as in the "flop-and-drop" type of knee-drop attack), the ballistic energy would go down into the mat. But if the attacker rotates his body so he corkscrews under his opponent, the ballistic energy (the torque) is increased. Knee-drop throwing attacks are popular because they are often more difficult to counter than other throwing attacks.

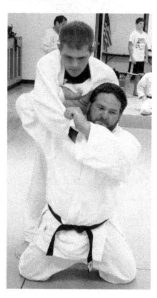

Flop-and-Drop Seoi Nage: If the attacker does a "flop-and-drop" knee-drop attack, the kinetic force and energy are expended directly down into the mat and wasted. The idea here is to throw an opponent over the attacker's body and onto the mat—not simply to drop down in front of him. In the 1960s and 1970s, when knee-drop attacks started to gain in popularity, people often did them flop-and-drop style. A negative outgrowth of these attacks was "negative judo." Athletes would use this type of attack if they were leading in the score and wanted to fool the referee into thinking they were actually trying to attack their opponent. In reality, they would be attempting to prevent their opponent from launching an attack and at the same time trying to run out the clock. As the contest rules changed to discourage this type of knee drop, athletes discovered the value of knee-drop throws, if done optimally using the corkscrew type of movement. As a result, knee-drop throwing attacks became more effective and are now considered viable throwing techniques.

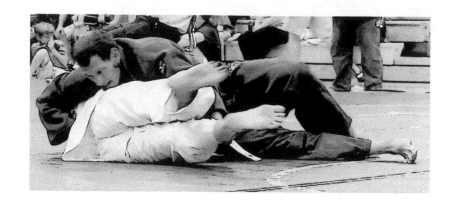

"Function dictates form."

—Louis Sullivan

CHAPTER 12

Generating Power

Generating Power

Power has been previously discussed in this book, including different ways of functionally applying it. This part of the book will examine the principles and biomechanical tools that generate power in judo.

Kinetic Energy: Kinetic energy is created by force generated by the attacker when throwing an opponent. As the attacker starts his movement with force and speed (power) and continues with the throwing attack, kinetic energy continues to build and eventually ends in a hard landing for the defender. The way to describe this kinetic building of energy is ballistics. As the attacker starts his movement with force and speed (remember that force and speed equal power), kinetic energy is formed. This kinetic energy travels through the attacker's body like links in a chain as it gains velocity and creates an explosive or ballistic effect. The ballistic force culminates in the release of this power as the attacker throws his opponent to the mat.

This initial force in kinetic energy has to start from somewhere and that "somewhere" is from the primary movers of the action—the human body's muscles.

It is important to point out that there is a difference between the application of kinetic energy in judo or other grappling sports and striking sports like boxing or karate. In a throwing technique in judo, the opponent's body is suspended or controlled by the actions of the attacker. There is less applied force behind a judo throwing technique than a punch in boxing. That's not to say that less force is initially generated by the judo athlete, but it does mean that the force generated by the judo athlete is directed so it lifts or suspends his opponent off the mat and at the same time, this generated force is used to control where and how an opponent is moved. The judo athlete isn't simply knocking his opponent down as a boxer would do with a punch. The boxer is concerned only with delivering the punch effectively, not how his opponent travels through the air or how the opponent lands on the mat. The judo athlete's concern is how his opponent travels through the air with as much control as possible and how hard he lands on the mat.

Compare a punch to an overhead press in weightlifting. A punch can deliver its generated power with more ballistic effect because it merely strikes an object. An overhead press, on the other hand, delivers less generated power because the lifter has to suspend and control the barbell during the lift. A punch doesn't have to hold or suspend any part of the body it strikes. No part of the kinetic effort is used to control the opponent. The punch just strikes. As a result, the ballistic effect is greater on impact. An athlete must suspend the barbell for several seconds, where the same force is generated and expended over a much shorter period of time in a punch. When an athlete lifts the barbell up and off his shoulders in the overhead press, he must control the movement of the bar. In both the overhead press and a throwing technique, some of the kinetic energy is expended in the suspending (or lifting or throwing) action of the movement. This is why optimal technical application (skill) is essential for both a weightlifter and a judo athlete.

Primary Movers: The primary movers are the main muscles of the body involved in any movement. Power comes from somewhere. It's not a mystical force but rather a biomechanical phenomenon the attacker generates. To apply power efficiently, the human body must be physically strong enough to generate it, especially under stressful conditions.

In a throwing technique such as seoi nage, where the attacker throws his opponent over his body and forward onto the mat, the attacker's primary movers are his legs and feet. By driving off his feet that are attached to the mat, he starts a power chain through his legs, into his hips and upper body, and eventually into and through his arms and hands, which are the points of contact with the defender's body. The power is focused in the direction of the attack and builds velocity as the attack continues.

Train for a "Fighter's Physique": This is why **specificity of strength** training is important. Specificity of strength means that an athlete trains and develops the muscles that are most commonly used in judo. Train to develop a "fighter's physique" rather than a bodybuilder's physique. Physical preparation (aerobic, nonaerobic, and range of motion/flexibility) is an integral and necessary aspect of a judo athlete's overall training program. Without a healthy, strong body, functional application of technical skill is not possible, especially under the stressful conditions of competition.

Limb Position: This is a term used in all sports. It means that using your hands, arms, legs, feet, and head in the most efficient way possible will make any technique more effective. The position of any part of the body determines how effectively it can be used. Every component of the body must work in a coordinated way for optimal efficiency and effectiveness. When some part of the body is not in the proper position, the technique being applied will not be as effective as it should be. The attacker will then have to modify the technique (if possible) to make up for the less-than-efficient placement of the limb or other body part.

Often, optimal limb position is based on the most effective use of the hips, which is dependent on the placement of the feet and legs. The more stable the base is, the more efficient the use of the limbs can be. Power is generated from the mat or floor up through the feet, the length of the leg, and then into the hip. From here, the rotational movement of the hip can increase the already generated force from the lower extremities up through the body, into the arms, and eventually into the hands that connect attacker and defender. For all of this to happen, the limbs must be positioned correctly. If, for example, your arm is in the wrong place at the wrong time, it could mess up your technique.

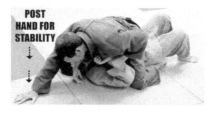

A good example of correct or incorrect limb placement is the use of the arms and hands in a pinning technique to distribute the attacker's body weight. The base of an osaekomi waza is fluid and moving, and the attacker continually shifts and moves to retain control of the defender. A major aspect of the shifting and moving to retain control is how the attacker uses his hands, arms, head, feet, legs, and knees to "post" (think of a post holding a fence solidly in the ground) on the mat to maintain balance and stability. As this photo shows, the attacker uses his extended right hand and arm to post onto the mat for stability, allowing himself to reposition his body weight as necessary to maintain the osaekomi waza.

Speed of Entry: This is how fast, and in which direction, the attack is made. A more accurate way of describing this action would be "velocity of entry" but "speed of entry" is more commonly used. Both static foot-speed drills and moving foot-speed drills are essential for developing an athlete's speed of entry into a throwing technique.

Ballistic: This is the launching and flight of any object. Usually associated with the study of rockets and bullets, ballistics also takes into consideration other things that can be propelled, slung, or thrown such as a baseball. In other words, it is the effect of an object (for our purpose, a human body) moving with speed in relation to the force of gravity through the air.

Ballistic Object: This describes any projectile, body, or object in flight. In judo, the human body is a ballistic object. When an athlete throws his opponent to the mat, a ballistic effect takes place. As the defender's body is thrown and goes through the air, kinetic energy is built up. Traveling through the air, the defender's body picks up speed and creates energy. When the defender's body lands on the mat, what is created is ballistic effect.

Ballistic Effect: This des-cribes the action produced when a ballistic object hits its target (such as when a human body hits a mat). The more power behind putting an object into flight, the more ballistic force 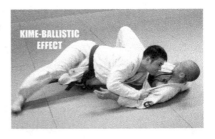 it will have and the more ballistic effect it will have when it hits another object. A good example is how hard an athlete's body lands on the mat when he has been thrown. The more force generated by the attacker into the throwing movement, the faster and harder the defender will hit the mat. This is known as **kime** in judo. Kime is the deciding or finishing action. The word means "to decide" and signifies the end result—the finish of a throwing technique. So, for our purposes, ballistic effect is force in relation to throwing an opponent to the mat. Kime is the ballistic force and describes how hard the defender hits the mat when thrown.

Throw: A throw is a ballistic action. It is one method of propelling something through the air. A baseball pitcher throws a baseball and a judo athlete throws his opponent. The judo term **nage** means "to throw, cast, project, or fling." A good example is seoi nage. "Seoi" means to "carry over the back" and "nage" means "throw" so the name of this technique describes what actually takes place.

Control: This means manipulating an opponent to control how, where, and when he can move. In other words, the attacker dictates how, where, and when the defender moves.

Force: Biomechanically, force equals mass times acceleration. This is a push, pull, or other movement that changes the state of motion of the defender's body. Force is the power generated by the attacker (power results from speed, strength, and acceleration). Force is necessary to move an object (for our purposes, a human body). Overcoming the defender's resting inertia requires force. What causes this to happen is known as **action force.** An action force is the force that acts in one direction when an athlete pushes off his foot (or both feet) in a throwing attack, or when he pushes off his feet in a groundfighting attack. When he does this, he exerts force into the ground and pushes off it. This driving off the feet is caused by **muscle force**, which is created when the muscles contract or are stretched. Newton's Third Law (which we saw earlier in this book) explains why the mat provides the **reaction force** necessary to execute a successful throwing technique.

Think about an attacker driving off his foot as he starts his throwing technique. His foot presses against the mat, driving downward and back against it. The force of this driving foot acts against the mat. However, as the attacker moves, gravity pulls the attacker's foot down and, as a result, the force pushes up against that driving foot. This answers why the attacker's body moves into the direction of the throw. The attacker moves because the action force of the attacker's foot against the mat creates a reaction force of the mat against his foot. An analogy is what takes place when a sprinter drives off the starting block. This explosive force drives the sprinter in the direction he wants to go. The action force created by the attacker when driving off his foot against the mat is reacted to by the reaction force of the mat, and this causes the attacker to move in the direction of the throwing action.

Force can also be seen as the result of the falling action of the human body. The amount of force created is directly related to how hard or how soft the body falls when thrown. How hard or how soft a person lands on the mat is directly related to the force that put him there. This is the **contact force** found in two primary instances. The first is when the attacker's and the defender's bodies first make contact. The second is when the defender's body makes contact with the mat. When the attacker throws his opponent onto the mat with **control and force**, ippon is awarded. These are the two primary criteria for what is considered in judo to be the ultimate display of technical skill, the **ippon**.

Why the Ippon Is Important in Judo: At this point, it might be interesting to discuss why an "ippon" is so important in judo. An ippon results when both control and power are exhibited in a technique. This is mostly thought to apply to throwing techniques, but it includes all technical skills (ask anyone who has been strangled or armlocked if there was control and force applied!). However, the results of control and power are usually most evident in a throwing technique. A look at the contest rules of judo through the years will show an ippon has always been achieved when one athlete throws his opponent with control and force—or in the case of groundfighting, when one athlete controls his opponent and applies force in such a way that the opponent is strangled, armlocked, or held for time in a pin. Another way of saying that a throw is finished with control and force is that it is finished with ballistic effect. This is why when training in throwing techniques, it is important to always achieve the most control and force possible. This is why the ippon is considered to be the ultimate goal of a judo contest.

Trajectory: We often think of rockets when it comes to trajectory, but for our purposes trajectory describes the flight path of the human body when it is thrown from a stable base on the mat. The trajectory of a human body depends on velocity (speed plus controlled direction). In some throwing techniques, the trajectory is minimal, such as with a foot sweep like okuri ashi barai or a low knee-drop seoi nage. In other cases, the trajectory is steep with a high-amplitude throw such as ura nage, the rear throw used in judo and sambo that lifts the defender up into the air and back down onto the mat with force and control.

Trajectory does not describe how fast the human body moves through the air but rather the angle at which it does so. This trajectory is based on the velocity of each specific throwing technique. The less lift vertically that takes place, the lower the trajectory, and the more lift vertically, the higher the trajectory. In other words, the higher the defender is thrown, the longer he stays in the air.

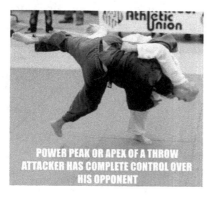

POWER PEAK OR APEX OF A THROW
ATTACKER HAS COMPLETE CONTROL OVER
HIS OPPONENT

Power Peak: This is the apex or pinnacle of a throwing technique. It is the highest point in the trajectory (flight path) of the body when it is thrown. This is the instant the defender's body changes directions in its course through the air. What goes up must come down, and the power peak describes the instant when this takes place.

Angle of Attack: This is the angle of the attacker's body in relation to the defender's body and how the throwing action develops into the trajectory as the throw accelerates. In throwing techniques where the defender's body is thrown over the attacker's body, a smaller, more compact, and rounder angle of attack is often the norm. This is true in throws such as uchi mata and seoi nage. In foot sweeps such as okuri ashi barai or in leg hooks or reaps such as o soto gari, the angle of attack is more linear and not as rounded or compact as in throws done over the attacker's body, as in seoi nage. In pick-up or lifting throws such as ura nage, where the defender is lifted up and off the mat, the trajectory and angle of attack is higher and linear at the start of the throw and becomes rounder at the power peak of the throw.

In other words, the attacker does not pick up his opponent straight into the air and throw him back down along the same trajectory. Instead, there is a rounder throwing action where the attacker throws his opponent over some part of his body. The uchi mata shown in this photo resulted in an ippon because of (among other reasons) the attacker's low, compact angle of attack. The angle of attack is one thing that makes the throwing techniques of judo effective. And as discussed elsewhere in this book, the attacker's rounded and rotational movement creates such torque and velocity that it makes it difficult for someone to escape a throwing attack.

In the next chapter, we will take a look at how, by "staying round," the attacker better controls the angle of attack, and the rotational movement that creates torque is more effectively applied. Let's now take a look at staying round.

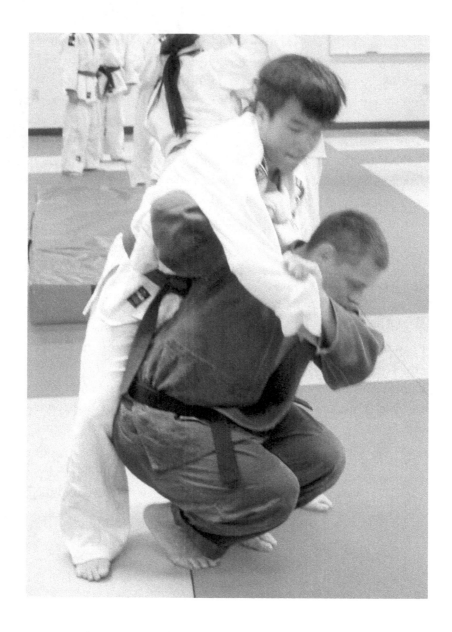

*"Throwing is the easy part. Getting into position every
time is the hard part."*

—Jerry Swett

CHAPTER 13

Staying Round

"Staying Round" and Using Rotation to Create Momentum

The concept of "staying round," or the use of rotational movement, is one of the principles that make judo so efficient. A judo skill is usually applied not in a straight line, but with a round, rotational movement. A throw, for example, does not go straight up and down but up and over the attacker's body in a rounded motion. Not all throwing techniques are rotational or rounded, but many are, and this is one of the common uses of movement in judo that make the activity so efficient from a biomechanical point of view.

The often-used word "nage" implies the idea of "throwing" or "projecting" the body of the defender, often over the attacker's body. Nage implies a controlled throwing of an object over another object (in this case, the attacker's body) and onto the mat. This use of rotational movement and the resulting momentum requires less physical strength to initiate and sustain the throwing movement. Take, for instance, a throw like tomoe nage. The attacker does not lift the defender straight up into the air and off the mat in a straight line. Instead he lifts him off the mat by tucking and rounding his body and going under the defender's center of gravity. Think of it as a wheel that the defender will roll over. The rotational or wheeling action rolls and throws the defender up and over the attacker's body. "Staying round" allows more momentum and ballistic effect in the throwing action.

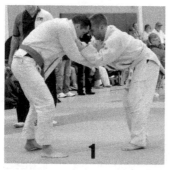

1. This first photo shows the attacker (on the right) using the combined effects of controlling the space between himself and his opponent and controlling the posture through gripping to force his opponent to start to bend forward in order to set him up for the throw to follow.

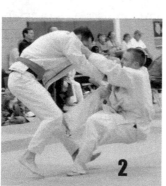

2. The attacker tucks and curls his body, making it round as he swings the lower part of his body in and under his opponent's center of gravity. The attacker generates power from his left foot, which is driving off the mat.

3. The attacker has successfully tucked and gone under the defender's center of gravity. The attacker continues to drive off his left foot to generate power into the throwing action. The momentum continues to build until the apex of the throwing action.

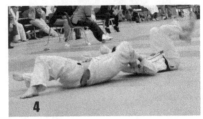

4. The attacker has successfully thrown his opponent with tomoe nage with control and force, scoring ippon.

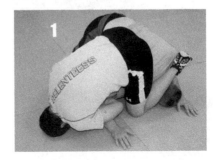

Staying Round in Newaza

The ability to stay round isn't limited to throwing techniques or standing judo. It is used just as effectively in newaza (groundfighting). In fact, the newaza of judo is based on this fluid, rotational, and "round" approach.

There are a lot of examples of how judo groundfighting emphasizes staying round, but a commonly used one is rolling an opponent over from a stable to an unstable position. These turnovers or breakdowns are similar to throwing techniques. Instead of starting from a standing position, they begin with both athletes engaged in groundfighting. For the purposes of our discussion, let's first use juji gatame, the cross-body armlock, as an example.

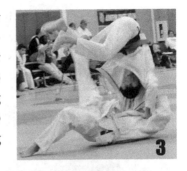

1. The attacker gains initial control over the defender as shown. Look at how the attacker's body is rounded and not

extended out in a straight line. The attacker positions his body in a stable way by using the top of his head for a base, thus allowing him to round his body as shown.

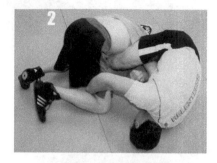

2. The attacker rolls to his left side, and by staying tucked and rounded, he generates more power and momentum for the rolling action. The attacker's goal is to roll the defender over and onto his back.

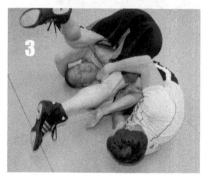

3. This shows the attacker and defender midway through the rolling action. The attacker uses his hands and arms to trap the defender's arm and leg to gain control and better roll his opponent. This rolling, rotary action is swift, and the momentum increases as the roll continues. The defender is now being forced to roll over his head and shoulders and will land on his back.

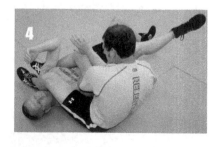

4. The attacker has successfully rolled the defender over and onto his back. The attacker now controls his opponent in a leg-press position and uses his hands and arms to continue to trap the defender's right arm to the attacker's torso. This trap-

ping action allows the attacker to add even more momentum to this movement when he rolls back to stretch the defender's arm straight.

5. The attacker has success-fully rolled his opponent over and onto his back, trapping the defender's right arm and rolling back to lever the arm out straight to apply the juji gatame.

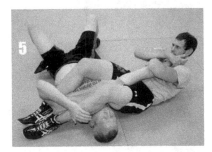

This roll into juji gatame is an example of the attacker "staying round" and forcing his oppo-nent to do the same.

Here is another example of staying round in newaza. In this case, the attacker is using a turnover or breakdown against an opponent positioned on all fours and will turn him over and onto his back to apply an osaekomi waza (pinning technique).

In this breakdown or turnover sequence, the attacker forces his opponent to "stay round" and as a result turns the defender onto his back for an osaekomi waza. The attacker also uses the concept of "shiho," or controlling the defender's four corners, that will be explained a bit later. This is a standard far-arm, near-leg breakdown but is one of those biomechanically sound skills that work at all levels of competition.

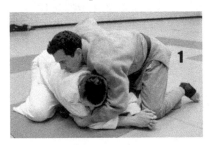

1. In this first photo, the defender is on all fours and the attacker is positioned at the defender's side. The attacker uses his left hand and arm to trap and pull in on the defend-er's right elbow.

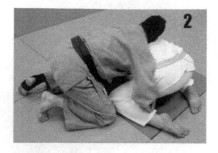

2. This view shows how the attacker uses his right hand and arm to trap and control the defender's left upper leg and hip area.

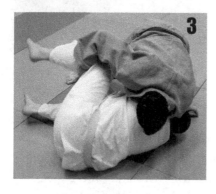

3. The attacker uses his left hand and arm to pull in on the defender's right elbow and uses his right hand and arm to lift the defender's left leg. This action rolls the defender over the defender's right shoulder as shown.

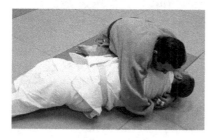

4. The attacker has turned his opponent over onto his back and secures the mune gatame (chest hold).

This example shows how the attacker can use the concept of staying round against an opponent by forcing the opponent to be round in order to turn him over and onto his back.

Staying Round in Bottom Newaza: When fighting off the buttocks or hips in the bottom position, staying round provides more freedom of movement than if the athlete is flat on his back or linear. This mobility permits the athlete to initiate more attacks and be more aggressive from the bottom position.

1. This photo sequence starts with the bottom athlete, the attacker, on his buttocks with his feet inside his opponent's legs for control. The attacker uses an arm drag to start his move to get his opponent's back.

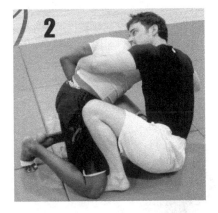

2. The attacker improves his position by working to his opponent's right side and starting to get control of the opponent's back using his left hand to control the opponent's left hip. The attacker uses his left hand on his opponent's hip to pull himself up and onto his opponent's back.

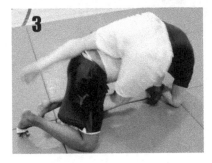

3. The attacker is now on his opponent's back and drives his right foot and leg under his opponent's right hip and upper leg. The attacker swings his left leg over the bottom athlete's left hip.

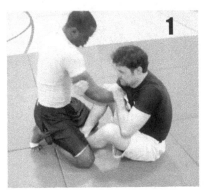

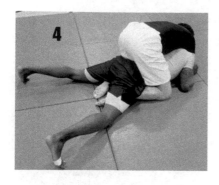

4. The attacker secures both of his feet and legs in his opponent's hips and upper legs for control in this rodeo ride. Then the attacker flattens his opponent in order to apply a choke.

Fighting off the bottom in this way is called **newaza no semekata** (attack form in fighting off the buttocks) and is most effective when the bottom athlete is round and positioned on his buttocks or hips rather than flat on his back.

The defining characteristics of judo groundfighting are its fluidity and fast pace. This fluidity is based on efficient and economical movement that depends less on strength and more on controlling movement. All of this comes from the fact that judo athletes generally stay round in their movements. This round, rotational-based movement produces more torque in the application of submission techniques.

Let's now look at another biomechanical concept that explains why judo works: the four corners of the human body.

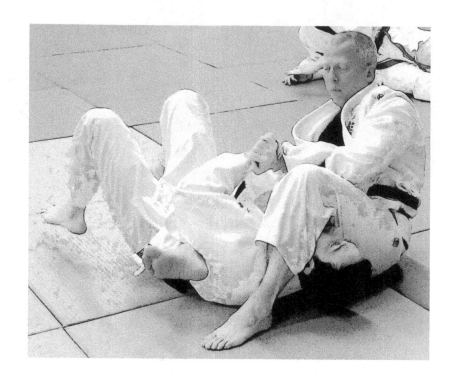

"One of the worst places to be is flat on your back looking up at the ceiling lights with an opponent pinning you."

—Ken Brink

CHAPTER 14

Shiho: The Four Corners of the Body

Shiho: The Four Corners of the Body

The concept of "shiho" or "four corners" describes the major controlling points of the human body. The use of these points was initially developed in judo as a practical method of control. These four corners are the two shoulders and the two hips. While there are certainly other parts of the body that can (and are) used to control an opponent, controlling one or both of the opponent's shoulders and hips works with a high degree of success. This is because the concept is based on sound biomechanical principles.

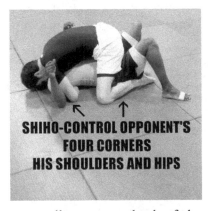

SHIHO-CONTROL OPPONENT'S FOUR CORNERS HIS SHOULDERS AND HIPS

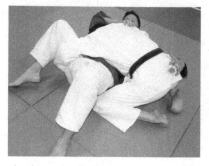

One of the first pinning techniques that come to mind when talking about "shiho" is yoko shiho gatame (side four corner hold). This side control position permits the attacker to optimally control his opponent at both the shoulder area and the hip area. The attacker can adjust his base with his hips and legs to effectively control his opponent for an extended length of time.

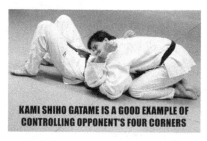

KAMI SHIHO GATAME IS A GOOD EXAMPLE OF CONTROLLING OPPONENT'S FOUR CORNERS

Kami shiho gatame (upper four corner hold), yoko shiho gatame (side four corner hold), and tate shiho gatame (vertical four corner hold) are three of the most fundamental osaekomi waza (pinning or immobilization techniques) and are all based on the concept of "shiho." While there are other effective osaekomi waza, these three form a central core of technical skill in judo.

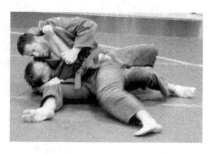

Some pins that may seem to not be based on the concept of shiho are very much dependent on this biomechanical principle. A good example is kesa gatame (scarf hold or pin). On the surface, it looks like a "head and arm pin" as used in wrestling. However, looking at it more closely, as the attacker controls his opponent's head and right arm (as shown), he simultaneously controls the defender's right shoulder. By optimal placement of his legs and hips as his base, the attacker effectively controls the defender's right hip as well. By effective placement and use of his feet, legs, and hips, the attacker provides a stable yet fluid and moveable base to control his opponent.

Here is an example of sankaku gatame (triangle pin) where the attacker uses sankaku (triangle) control with the legs on her opponent's left shoulder, arm, and head. The attacker uses her left arm to grab and trap the defender's

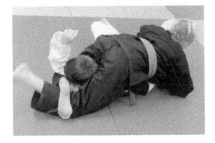

right hip and upper leg. This is a good example of how the attacker exerts control across the defender's body by controlling opposite corners of the defender's body (right shoulder and left hip).

Controlling an opponent's shoulders and hips is not limited to pinning techniques. Look at how the attacker (on top) controls his opponent's four corners in this rodeo ride.

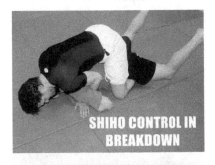

SHIHO CONTROL IN BREAKDOWN

1. Here is a commonly used groundfighting skill. We call this the "rodeo ride," a phrase I believe my friend John Saylor was the first to use back in the early 1980s. The attacker gains control of his opponent and gets his back as shown. Look at

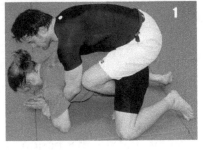

how the attacker's feet and legs are dug in to control the defender's hips and lower body. The attacker uses his hands and arms to hook under the defender's shoulders to start the process of controlling his upper body as well.

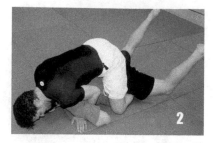

2. As the attacker drives his body forward, he sinks his feet and legs in more deeply at the defender's hips to exert even more control of the lower body. The attacker uses both hands and arms to trap the defender's arms and shoulders. This drives the defender forward and flat onto his front.

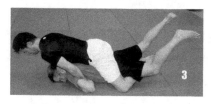

3. The attacker continues to drive forward and in a "rocking" movement forces the defender's hips and legs upward and the defender's shoulders and upper body forward. The attacker has control of the defender's four corners and is in complete control of the situation. The attacker can now proceed to a choke or other technique.

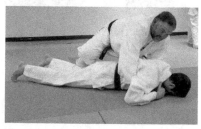

Utsubuse: This term means "hiding on the front" and is a fairly common position in judo. The contest rules in judo are lenient in this situation, allowing limited time to engage in newaza. As a result of this, this utsubuse position is used tactically as a way to stall long enough and wait for the referee to call a halt to the action in order for the bottom athlete to get out of the situation. However, if the top athlete can demonstrate to the referee that he can gain a controlling position and use that position to effectively work for a submission technique or a turnover for a pin, the action will be permitted to continue. This is a risky tactic on the bottom athlete's part as he is vulnerable to having his opponent gain control over his hips as well as his shoulders and arms as shown in the next photo.

The top athlete has control over the opponent's hips with his legs and the opponent's shoulders and arms with his arms and hands. So the four corners of the bottom grappler are being controlled in this rodeo ride. An obvious and often-used attack the top athlete can use from this position is a hadaka jime (naked choke).

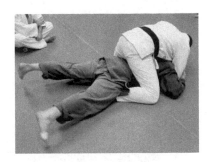

Aomuke: This word means being supine or face up. The bottom athlete in this photo is in the aomuke position. The controlling athlete is using what is called a leg press but is also referred to as the "juji gatame position." Whatever the name, the fact is that the bottom athlete is in trouble. This,

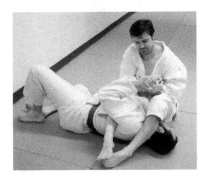

like the utsubuse position, is a defensive position. The top athlete controls the four corners of his opponent's body and has both time and opportunity to secure a juji gatame (cross-body armlock) or switch to another technique such as uki gatame (straddle hold) or sankaku jime (triangle strangle).

Controlling an opponent's hips or shoulders does not always require grabbing the opponent. The top athlete uses his hand to "check" or control his opponent's near hip by placing it on the mat and will move it as necessary to

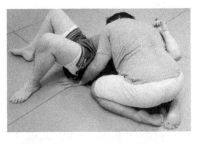

maintain control. The top athlete has good control over his opponent's head and shoulders in this variation of mune gatame (chest hold) and yoko shiho gatame (side four corner hold).

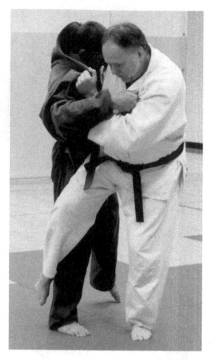

Controlling the four corners isn't confined only to ground-fighting. It has relevance in throwing techniques as well. By controlling an opponent's shoulders, the attacker can "steer" the defender's body in the same way he would use a steering wheel on a car. When you control an opponent's shoulders, you control his hips as well—and when you control both his hips and shoulders, you will control his movement.

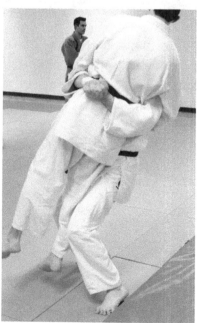

In this photo, the attacker controls his opponent's hips in lifting his opponent in a variation of ura nage, the rear throw. There are numerous ways to control an opponent's hips and entire hip area, both outside the hips and grabbing or reaching between the opponent's legs in throwing techniques. This controlling action is called a "tight-waist" for an obvious reason: the attacker is holding his opponent's waist tightly.

An often-used example of how an athlete controls his opponent's hips is when he limits or nullifies his opponent's hips as a defensive move using taisabaki such as a hip block as shown here. In this case, the defender (on the left in this photo) turns his hips and drives his near (left) hip into the attacking (right) hip of his opponent. This action negates the throwing movement and stops the 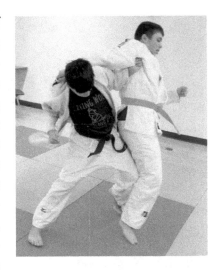 opponent's forward momentum in the throwing attack.

Controlling the four corners of the human body is an integral concept in all aspects of judo movement. This is especially true in defensive movement as will be examined in the next chapter.

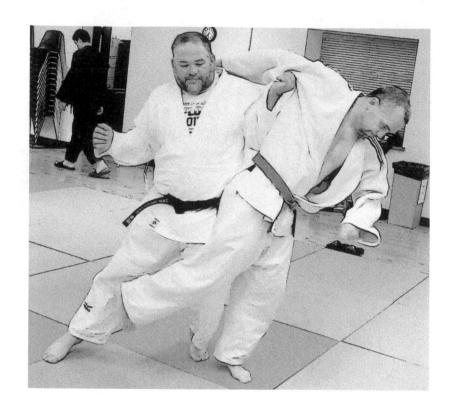

*"Attack and defense are one in the same depending
on the situation."*

—Definition of Kobo Ichi

CHAPTER 15

Using Movement in Defense

Using Movement in Defense

So far, this book has focused primarily on controlling movement for the application of offensive skills. But of course controlling movement applies to defensive skills as well. While there are numerous specific skills designed to block, evade, avoid, or negate an opponent's attack, there are some generic and overarching principles that translate to movement patterns in defensive skills. Defensive skills are integral to any grappling sport but especially to judo because of its technically complex and advanced throwing techniques. As my good friend John Saylor often says, "A good part of winning is not getting beat." What he means is that if you can defend yourself and stay competitive, there's always the possibility of gaining the advantage and beating your opponent.

Identifying and Examining Various Biomechanical Defensive Movements

There are numerous specific defensive and escape movements that comprise what can be called "lines of defense" similar to a defensive perimeter in the military. These lines of defense are detailed in my earlier book *Winning on the Mat*. But analyzing the overall biomechanics involved in applying defensive skills against throwing techniques reveals five primary and generic movements. These five are as follows: 1. prevent, 2. hip block, 3. evade, 4. avoid, and 5. turn out. There are many applications and variations of each, but these five provide a structure for the teaching and learning of defensive skills.

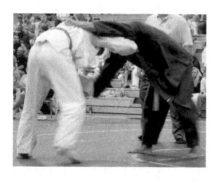

Prevent by Use of Grip and Posture: Often an attack can be stopped in its tracks by the defender's gripping and posture. This is a subtle form of offensive and defensive movement. The athlete with the dominant grip and superior posture will many times be considered the attacker. In grip-fighting sequences, the give and take of gripping action changes the offense and defense for each athlete. This is a good example of kobo ichi, which will be defined later. An examination of each phase of preventive defensive skill follows. Grip fighting is the first phase of keeping an opponent at bay. Both offensive and defensive gripping skills are used to put an opponent into position so he can't attack effectively. In very real terms, using gripping as a means of defense is actually "preventive" defense, and thus the name for this aspect of defense. In other words, it is shutting your opponent down as much as possible with good grip fighting so he can't launch an attack against you. Just as in medicine, an ounce of prevention is worth a pound of cure. The second phase of preventive defensive skills is body movement and control of the opponent's posture. This includes an effective use of body space; in other words, how close or far you are from your opponent. Jigotai (defensive posture) has a valid use in this aspect of defense. Every athlete makes use of jigotai. However, the excessive use of a defensive posture leads to passive judo. If an athlete's only concern is to keep from being thrown without any regard to putting himself in position for a counterattack, he will make jigotai his primary posture. The best advice in using jigotai is to use it when necessary—and only when necessary. To sum it up, making sure that you are in a position so your opponent can't effectively attack by your use of posture, grip, or how fast you move about the mat is an effective defensive skill.

Hip Block and Cut Away 1: This is the hip block and cut away defense. This type of defense literally stops the forward momentum of the attacker's throwing action. In this defensive action, the defender's explosive hip rotation creates the torque that counteracts and negates the attacker's throwing 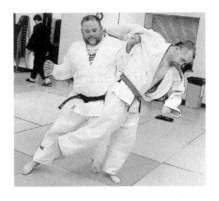 action. This hip rotation is one form of **taisabaki**. This defense has a high ratio of success, as it not only stops the attacker's momentum, but because the attacker's inertia is abruptly ended, the attacker has more time to launch his counterattack. In the photo above, the defender (left) does a hip block and cut away against the attacker's uchi mata. Look at how the defender uses his left hand to push away and steer the attacker's upper body.

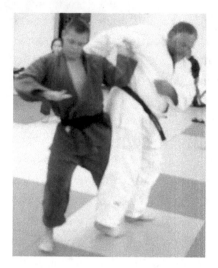

Hip Block and Cut Away 2: Here is a basic application of the hip block and cut away. Using the hips to block an attack is one of the most effective methods of stopping a throw, especially a forward throw. The strong rotational action of the defender's hips impacts the attacker's hips and stops his momentum. This is good use of taisabaki or hip turning action. In the hip block, the defender will use his left hip to block, or jam, his opponent's right-sided throwing attack. From this, the defender stops the momentum of the forward-throwing attack and regains his balance to reestablish himself as a threat to his opponent. Basically, you cut with your opposite hip, hit him hard with that hip, and don't let your opponent get past your hip. Not permitting an attacker to get past the hip is a key element in defense, and it is actually often said, "Don't let your opponent get past your hips." If the attacker does get past (or on the inside) of the defender's hips, the attacker will have a much better chance of throwing the defender. If the attacker slips his hip in, he can still catch the defender in a throw, so the defender must block his attack hard. The defender should also "cut away" from the attack if possible. As the defender blocks with his left hip, he must tear his right hand away from the attacker's grasp and maybe even step back a bit with his right leg and foot. In this photo, the defender's (left in photo) effective use of taisabaki as a hip-turning action negates the forward momentum and stops the attacker's throw. As he does this, the defender pulls his right arm away and jams his left hand and arm into the side of the attacker. This action helps in stopping the forward momentum of the attack and will be used to give the defender the space and time to launch his counterattack.

Hip Block and Cut Away 3: This view from the rear shows how the defender rotates his hips, generating the force to stop the attacker's forward direction. To add power to the torque of the hip movement, the defender steps back and away with his right foot and uses it as a stable base. The hip block is a

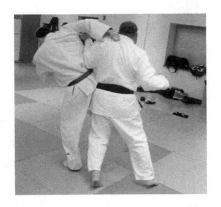

popular and effective defensive movement because it has a high rate of success and permits the defender the opportunity to launch his counterattack.

Evade Attack by Hopping Around: As the attacker launches his throw, the defender will either hop back or around the attacker's hips and body to evade the throwing action. This photo shows the defender (left) hopping around to his left to evade this tai otoshi attack. This defense is used primarily against forward throws such as tai otoshi, seoi nage, or uchi mata but can be used against any

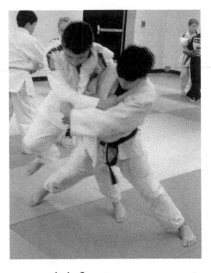

forward-throwing attack. The hop-around defensive movement is one of the most often used forms of defense in judo.

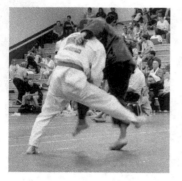

Evade Attack by Cutting against the Grain: In evading the throw, the defender may shift the direction of his body behind his attacker's direction of attack. This is "cutting against the grain" (or direction) of the attacker's throw by moving behind the attacker. Instead of hopping around the outside of the attacker in a circular movement, the defender cuts behind the attacker in a linear direction. This photo shows the defender (left) evading the uchi mata attack by cutting against the direction of the throw. As he does this, the defender grabs the attacker's left leg to set up a counterthrow. Grabbing the leg is not part of this evading action but is shown in this photo to illustrate how quickly a defensive action can turn into an offensive (counterattack) action. While grabbing the leg is not currently permitted in International Judo Federation (IJF) contest rules, it is permissible in the rules of other judo organizations such as the Amateur Athletic Union (AAU) as well as in sambo, BJJ, and sport jujitsu.

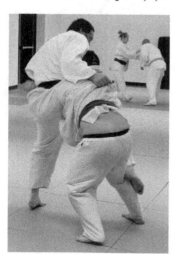

Evade by Sprawling or Bagging Out: The defender may also evade the attack by lowering the level of his body, bending forward to get his hips as far away from the attacker as possible, and moving directly to his rear by "bagging out." The defender does this in an effort to create as much space as possible between himself and the attacker. This photo shows an example of this. Another example would be to "sprawl" backward to avoid an opponent's morote gari, or double leg takedown.

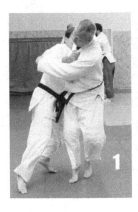
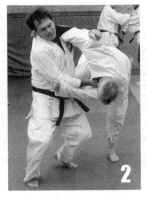
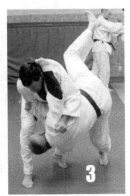

Avoid: What is called **sukashi** (meaning "to avoid") is an effective defensive movement that places the defender in good position to immediately launch his counterattack. The sukashi action is a commonly used defense against an uchi mata attack. In this photo sequence, the defender uses the sukashi movement to avoid and then counter his opponent.

At this point, it should be mentioned that four of these defensive movements (excluding the turn out) could be considered functional applications of **kuzushi** (in addition to **happo no kuzushi** and **hando no kuzushi**). Performing these defensive movements can, and often does, control the movement and balance of the attacker so the kaeshi waza can be applied.

Turn Out: This is the last-ditch effort on the part of the defender to prevent himself from landing on his back or side by turning out of the throw in mid-air. An important element in this method is to have the mental and physical wherewithal to use it when needed. This is the least recommended defense and should be done only by skilled, elite athletes

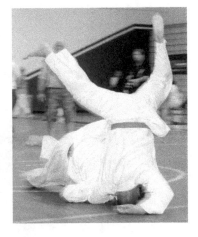

who have excellent kinesthetic awareness. *Important:* Under no circumstances should an athlete or student ever—and I mean *ever*—land in a bridge position when thrown on the back. Landing in a bridge position to avoid landing on the back is extremely dangerous and could result in a broken neck or other serious injuries.

Kaeshi Waza: Counter techniques are the actions applied in both standing and groundfighting situations where the defender blocks, nullifies, evades, or avoids the attack of his opponent and counters with his own technique. Kaeshi translates to "reversal of direction or in a counter direction" and waza translates to "technique." It's safe to say that every action has an opposite reaction, and this is the functional theory behind kaeshi waza. This photo series shows ura nage (rear throw), which is a commonly used counter throw against an opponent's forward-throwing attack. In this application, the defender (on the right) has lowered the level of his body and shifted behind the attacker to cut against the grain of the throw. As he shifts his right hip behind his opponent, the defender now launches his counterattack as he lifts his opponent and rotates his body to his right and into the direction of his counter throw. The attacker finishes the throwing action by turning onto his opponent as he lands.

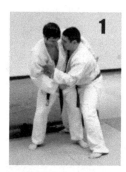 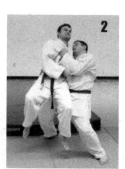 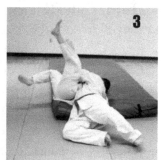

The Principles of Defensive Movement

Tactically, there are three primary defensive principles and an over-arching principle of attack and defense that form the framework for defensive movement or, more correctly stated, reactionary movement in judo. These principles apply in all aspects of judo technical movement, both standing and groundfighting. While these principles are used in judo, they (or variations of them) are fundamental principles also used in aikido, kendo, and other Japanese martial arts.

1. Go no Sen: Simply put, wait for your opponent's attack and use his movement against him. In Miyomoto Musashi's *The Book of Five Rings*, this is called **tai no sen**. This is different than a counterattack where you, as the defender, stop his offensive action by blocking, avoiding, or evading it and then counter with your own attack.

2. Sen (Also Called Sen Sen no Sen): Your actions and movement negate your opponent's upcoming offensive technique. You, as the defender, anticipate his movement and deny him the opportunity or ability to initiate his attack. In other words, by reading his body movement, you stop him before he starts. Be at the right place at the right time, and take the initiative to get the better position under the circumstances.

3. Tai Tai no Sen: This is a simultaneous attack and your technique is the one that scores.

4. Kobo Ichi: A concept referenced by Donn Draeger in his excellent (and highly recommended) book *Modern Bujutsu and Budo* is kobo ichi. This principle is often used in judo and is best described as an "aggressive defense."

Kobo ichi is an old Japanese military and martial arts concept that attack and defense are one in the same. Which has priority depends on the situation. This is a fluid offense-defense where an athlete can, and will, turn a defensive situation into an offensive one depending on the situation. It is a state of mind as well as a physical act. "Kobo" means "attack (ko) and defense (bo)." "Ichi" implies "one or the same thing." In other words, offense and defense are part of the same action and will interchange as necessary. What this means in practical terms is that if an athlete views the time he has to defend himself as an opportunity to turn the attack around and beat his opponent, he has an advantage. This strategic attitude plays itself out in what can be best described as an "aggressive defense." When an athlete knows he can quickly turn a defensive action into an offensive action, this gives him a definite psychological edge. This is an integral aspect of controlling an opponent's movement and means constantly trying to place yourself in a good position and your opponent in a bad position. A good defense doesn't happen overnight. It takes work. Defensive skills should be practiced on a regular basis.

Conclusion

When Shawn Watson was nine years old, he came up to me at judo practice one evening and said, "Hey, this judo stuff works!" He explained how he used judo to quickly end a fight with a neighborhood bully (Shawn threw the kid with o soto gari) and said how he couldn't wait to learn more. Shawn went on to become a skilled and successful athlete at the national and international levels as well as an excellent coach. And he was right: this judo stuff does work. The purpose of this book has been to explain why and how it works.

If we understand why and how the human body moves, we will better appreciate how that movement can be used to form the basic structures of judo's many techniques. Whether we are athletes or coaches, we will be better able to appreciate the many functions these techniques are capable of having. When that is achieved, we will be better able to adapt these basic forms to make them functional skills with a high rate of success against fit, skilled, and motivated competition. This book has been about why a judo movement or technique works, how it works from a basic biomechanical perspective, and then how to make that technique work for the individual actually doing it.

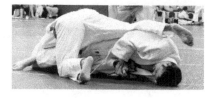 It is difficult enough for an athlete to control his or her own movement, but in judo, an athlete has to not only control what he does and how he moves but what his opponent does and how he moves. It's a well-known fact that it takes two people to make a throw happen. One person will initiate and the other will react. What happens next largely depends on the skill of the two contestants and how they interact with each other. Think of nonconfrontational sports: track and field, downhill skiing, or weightlifting. These athletes compete *with* each other to be the fastest, strongest, and the most skilled. In combat sports such as judo, by contrast, athletes compete *against* each other, and there is a difference in the dynamics of what goes on.

The consequences in judo for not effectively controlling an opponent include getting thrown to the mat, getting an arm stretched or cranked, being choked, and being held on the back for time—and getting a good look at the ceiling. Sports like football or rugby are tough games, but they are team sports and, ultimately, they are games. The goal is to get the ball into the end zone. Additionally, if a player makes a mistake, his teammates may be able to compensate for it. Team sports are good about teaching how to work as a unit, but in judo, there is no team to rely on, and the purpose of the sport isn't to get a ball into an end zone, but rather to throw, pin, or force an opponent to submit from a submission technique. As a result, it's more personal because there is more personal risk invested by the athlete— physically, mentally, and emotionally. Controlling the movement of another human being who is actively attempting to do the same thing to you is difficult due to the stress of this more personal type of competition.

This book has focused on the physical aspect of judo, and specifically, the controlling of movement based on rational mechanical principles in a realistic and competitive setting. But it must be said again that Kodokan judo has a much broader scope and purpose than merely winning judo matches. Early in judo's history, Professor Kano developed what he called the "three culture principle" for judo, an underlying principle that continues to have relevance today. This principle has three applicable tenets: 1. rentai-ho (judo as physical education and the development of a healthy body), 2. shobu-ho (skill in contests or self-defense), and 3. shushin-ho (good moral virtue and character development). Based on these three principles, judo is more than simply a sport. As I said in this book's introduction, judo as a sport is based on judo as a method of physical education.

As an author and coach, I have attempted to provide a rational explanation of the basic biomechanical movements and technical applications of the very complex and compelling sport of judo. I hope what has been presented on the pages of this book will stimulate thought on the part of all who read it and compel them to delve into a more comprehensive study (and application) of technical skill and movement. It is with sincere humility and appreciation of the work by others that this book has been produced. As stated in this book's introduction, all books stand on the work of others, and this book is certainly no different. I have been fortunate to learn from many outstanding coaches, technicians, athletes, and authors through the years. It's my personal belief that coaches and serious students of judo should be in the habit of reading and studying as many sources of information as possible. There are a lot of great books out there. I hope you read them. This book is also intended to be a positive contribution to the existing body of knowledge on the science and art of teaching movement in the context of judo. The better we understand how the human body works and moves, and the better we know about how to make it work efficiently, the better we coaches will impart this to our students. As a result, both the athletes and judo in general will benefit.

ACKNOWLEDGMENTS

Special thanks to Sharon Vandenberg, Donna Bybee, and Joe Mace for many of the photographs in this book. Also, thanks to David Ripianzi, T. G. LaFredo, Barbara Langley, and all the YMAA team, with a special thanks to my patient and skilled editor, Doran Hunter. YMAA Publishing has been welcoming, supportive, friendly, and highly professional in the production of this book.

This book would not have been possible without the great cooperation of all the Welcome Mat coaches and athletes as well as coaches and athletes affiliated with our AAU and Judo Black Belt Association programs. I am honored to be associated with these fantastic people.

Most of all, my wife Becky has my heartfelt and eternal gratitude for not only sharing life with me for all of these years but also for her loyal support and encouragement.

GLOSSARY

acceleration. A body's rate of change in velocity.

action. The movement of a body in a directed or planned pattern.

agility. In judo, an athlete's ability to accelerate explosively and start a movement, decelerate (or even stop), and change direction then accelerate again in the new direction, maintaining control of both his body and his opponent's body with minimal reduction of speed.

ai yotsu. A stance that comes about when both athletes lead with the same-side hip and foot; in other words, a righty versus a righty.

anchor hand. The hand used to temporarily secure or "anchor" an opponent so the attacker can go on to gain more control with the other hand, change posture or stance, or move to further control of the situation. The anchor hand may or may not be the hand that makes initial contact with the opponent, but it is the hand that controls the opponent long enough to allow the attacker the opportunity to establish her position and stance.

apex. The power peak or highest point in a trajectory.

attacking leg. The leg (and foot) the attacker uses to control and manipulate the opponent's legs, feet, or body in the application of both throwing and groundfighting techniques.

automatic response. This takes place when the athlete's muscles have been taught how to perform a specific movement or skill without thinking about it first.

axis. An imaginary line passing through the body's (or any part of the body's) center of rotation. The center of any object (like a hub in a wheel).

ayumi ashi. A normal walking pattern. "Ayumi" means "walk" and "ashi" means "foot or leg." Together they imply the movement where the attacker and defender walk either forward or backward in a straight line.

balance. The ability of a body to maintain its control of equilibrium. See **equilibrium**.

ballistic. The launching and flight of any object and the effects of that launching or flight.

ballistic effect. The action produced when a ballistic object hits its target (for our purposes, a human body hitting a mat). The ballistic effect is the result produced by the ballistic action.

ballistic object. This describes any projectile, body, or object in flight.

base. The area of a body formed by the outermost points of contact with the mat. The base provides stability and optimal balance for the body.

biomechanics. The study of force and its effect on the human body.

block. The stabilizing object or agent that stops, limits, prevents, or controls the movement of a lever (for our purposes a lever would be an arm or leg).

breakdown. Taking an opponent from a stable to an unstable position in groundfighting. The best way to think about a breakdown is as a throwing technique in groundfighting. A breakdown can be applied from any starting position or posture and does not always turn an opponent over onto his back. See also **turnover**.

butsukari. A repetition drill to develop skill in throwing techniques. In butsukari, the emphasis is on the attacker's foot speed and tsurikomi action. The attacker enters into the technique but does not finish it by throwing his partner. This is also the older name for uchikomi, which is a similar drill, and not many people use the term butsukari today. However, the focus in uchikomi is a fast entry with emphasis on hip movement, and the focus in butsukari is foot speed and tsurikomi action. See also **uchikomi**.

center of gravity. The point where the weight of the body is concentrated. The point of the body where gravity is centered in all directions.

closed skill. A movement performed in a predictable pattern or in a controlled environment. The practice of nage no kata (form of throwing) is an example of a closed skill. Also called a closed-ended skill or movement.

contact force. The force resulting from two bodies touching each other.

control. Exerting influence over a body.

coupling. The connection of two parts in such a way that they work together as one unit. For our purposes, this takes place in the tsukuri phase of a technique where the attacker forms or builds the attack and fits his body into position to execute the technique.

debana. Instant of opportunity. This is the perfect timing of a technique's application.

direction of attack. The track of the movement the attacker establishes. There are eight angles or directions the body can travel in; the direction of attack may change from one angle to another or may remain constant.

direction of movement. The track or pattern established by a moving body. The direction of movement may change or remain constant.

drill training. Systematic and progressive use of movements and actions designed to teach and reinforce skill, fitness, and tactical ability. A drill is a systematic method of teaching using repeated movements and repetitions of specific actions.

driver leg. An integral part of the base of support in throwing and groundfighting techniques is the action of the driver leg. In most throws (as well as in groundfighting techniques), the attacker transfers power into the action by using his driver leg. This is also called the support leg. The driver leg not only provides a stable base, it is also used as a primary mover that generates power into the attacking movement. This is why it is called a "driver" leg: the attacker drives off it to initiate and continue his attack through to completion.

dynamics. The area of study concerned with rigid body mechanics and the accelerated motion of objects or bodies.

equilibrium. The state where there is neither acceleration nor deceleration. The ability of the body to maintain balance.

force. A pull or a push. Any influence that changes the state of motion of a body.

friction. The resistance or force caused by two surfaces moving or sliding against each other.

fulcrum. The axis or hinge about which the lever rotates.

gravity. The force of attraction between any two bodies.

hairi kata. Translates to "entry form" and is the generic name used in judo for the action of controlling movement when entering into a technique, usually a groundfighting technique.

hando no kuzushi. Hando means "reaction," no means "of," and kuzushi means "to break." This is one of two primary principles of control and of breaking the balance. In this principle, breaking balance is achieved by use of a diversionary movement. See also **happo no kuzushi.**

happo no kuzushi. Happo means "eight directions," no means "of," and kuzushi implies the breaking of balance. Happo no kuzushi are the eight directions in which a body can have its balance broken. They are 1. front, 2. back, 3. right side, 4. left side, 5. right front corner, 6. right rear corner, 7. left front corner, and 8. left rear corner. This method is a direct application of kuzushi where the attacker transmits direct force against the opponent's weak areas of balance. See also **hando no kuzushi**.

hikite. This is the pulling hand (also commonly called the sleeve hand). Hiki translates to "pull" and te translates to "hand."

impact. The collision between two bodies, or a body striking an object (as in a body hitting the mat when thrown).

inertia. A body's property of resisting inertia. It is the tendency of a body to stay at rest (not move) or to move continuously in a straight line at constant velocity.

instinctive response. An instinctive response is a natural or unconditioned reflexive action, and an automatic response is a learned or conditioned reflexive action.

ippon. The winning score in a judo contest. This word translates to "one point" and in this connection refers to a contest where the first score is the winner. The term is also used to imply "single" or "one point of an object" and is part of the names of techniques such as ippon seoi nage, or "one-armed shoulder throw." See also **seoi** and **waza-ari**.

jigotai. Defensive or bent-over posture. Jigo is "defensive" and tai is "posture of the body."

junbi-undo. Warm-up exercises.

kaeshi waza. Counterattacks where the defender blocks, nullifies, evades, or avoids the attack of his opponent and counters with his own technique. They are applied in both standing and groundfighting situations. Kaeshi translates to "reversal of direction or in a counter direction" and waza translates to "technique."

kake. The execution of the technique. The word kake can be translated as "suspend" and specifically refers to taking the opponent from his feet and putting him in the air, suspending and controlling his body in the process. This is the peak or apex of the throw or skill.

kansetsu waza. Translates to "joint techniques" and is used to describe all joint-locking techniques. Early in the twentieth century, the contest rules of judo were altered to allow locks only against the elbow joint.

kata. "Form" or "structure." Professor Kano developed several kata or prearranged forms starting in the early days of Kodokan judo's development in order to provide more structure to the training sessions and ensure that a standardized and skillful application of techniques be taught.

katame waza. The generic name used to describe all grappling and groundfighting techniques in judo. Katame means "holding something in place" and waza means "technique."

kenka yotsu. A stance formed when one athlete leads with his right side and his opponent leads with his left side. It is a righty-versus-lefty situation.

kime. "To finish" or "to decide." The term zanshin is also used to describe this finishing action of a throw. The word zanshin refers to "awareness" with the purpose of not relaxing but remaining focused during the final execution of a throwing technique. This is a sound concept, but I believe kime is more direct and equally sound as a way to describe what happens at the finish of a throwing technique. Think of kime as the follow-through or finish to the technique. This is the action that ensures the termination of the sequence of actions in the technique.

kinesiology. The study of human movement.

kinetic energy. Athletes' ability to perform work by virtue of their motion or movement or the motion of something else. Kinetic energy is created by force.

kobo ichi. This is an old Japanese military / martial arts concept that attack and defense are one in the same. Which has priority depends on the situation. This is a fluid offense-defense where an athlete can, and will, turn a defensive situation into an offensive one depending on the situation.

kodokan. "School to learn the way." This is the name Professor Jigoro Kano chose to describe his invention, judo. The Kodokan Judo Institute is located in Tokyo, Japan, and is considered the home of judo.

kowaza. Minor or "small" throwing techniques. These techniques are primarily foot and leg throws such as foot sweeps, reaps, or hooks such as okuri ashi barai and ko soto gari. Kowaza are not the large body throws such as uchi mata or tai otoshi. See also **owaza**.

kumi kata. The forms of grasping or gripping using jackets. The name is generically used to describe the gripping action. The word kumi means "grappling, or the action of two bodies engaged in a contest" and kata means "form."

kuzushi. The word kuzushi implies the breaking of balance and posture. Kuzushi is an important concept in the study, practice, application, and teaching of judo. Controlling the movement of an opponent and the ultimate breaking of his posture, stance, or balance is what makes all judo techniques efficient in their application.

lateral. Away from (at either side) the midline of the human body.

lead leg. Most athletes will lead with an extended hip, leg, and foot on one side or the other when they compete. This is often called the "lead leg." But in reality, the hip is what is leading, with the leg and foot positioned under it.

leg press. A controlling position also known as the "juji gatame position." The primary purpose of this position is to control an opponent in order to secure juji gatame (cross-body armlock), but it is not limited to the application of juji gatame and can also be used to secure different pinning or submission techniques.

lever. A barlike object that rotates around the axis of another object or body. The arm of the defender that is stretched across the pubic bone (serving as the fulcrum) of the attacker in the application of juji gatame (cross-body armlock) is an example.

limb position. The most efficient and effective placement and use of the hands, arms, legs, feet, and head. It is a term used in all sports.

line of force or **line of direction.** When the attacker uses his elbow to direct or aim where he will pull and steer his opponent, the direction of the movement of his elbow creates an imaginary line called the line of force (or line of direction). This line of force is created by the rotation of the attacker's body (creating torque) along with direct applied force from the attacker's deltoid muscle in his shoulder. Because of the way the shoulder, arm, and hand are biomechanically constructed, the attacker must always pull with his hand in the same direction that his elbow goes. In pulling, the hand follows the elbow. Conversely, in pushing, the movement of the elbow follows the movement of the hand.

linear. A straight line.

linear motion. The change in the position of the body (or any object) that takes place when all points of that body move in the same direction, the same distance, and at the same time.

makikomi. This is the result of an all-out throwing effort where the attacker throws his opponent to the mat and lands on him. This winding or rolling action is an extension of the kime or finishing action of a throw. Makikomi translates to "roll or wind one thing around or within another thing."

mass. The amount of matter or substance in a body. How much space the body takes up.

mechanics. The study of force and its effect on objects.

momentum. The speed of a body in movement. This is the mass of a body multiplied by its velocity. The larger the mass of an object, the larger the increase in momentum.

motion. Takes place when a body, or a part of a body, changes position.

motor skill. Any action that involves using muscles. Gross motor skills are larger movements of the muscles, and fine motor skills are smaller movements of the muscles.

movement. Controlled motion traveling in a specified direction. Movement takes place in a straight line, at an angular or circular direction, or a combination of both linear and angular.

movement time. This is the time it takes for a body to carry out a movement. See **reaction time**.

muscle memory. This is the same as motor learning, which involves integrating a specific motor task into memory through repetition. The more often an athlete practices a skill in an optimal way, the less time it takes for the brain to process how to do it, and therefore it becomes more automatic.

nage waza. This is the generic name for all throwing techniques in judo. Nage translates to "throwing, casting, or projecting," and waza translates to "technique."

newaza. A generic term used to describe groundwork or groundfighting. This is the name of one of the primary groundfighting positions developed in the early days of judo that continues to be used. See also **newaza no semekata**, **newaza shisei**, and **newaza shobu**.

newaza no semekata. "Forms of attack in groundfighting." This reclining position is the most basic position used for many years in Kodokan judo. Newaza translates to "reclining or supine technique." What is now called the guard is one of the oldest positions used in judo. Sumiyuki Kotani, Yoshimi Osawa, and Yuichi Hirose made specific reference to newaza no semekata (attacking forms of supine techniques) in their book *Newaza of Judo* published in 1973. Newaza no semekata describes the tactical and technical purpose of this position as primarily offensive. While defensive skills are initiated from this position, the intent is to attack.

newaza shisei. Posture in groundfighting.

newaza shobu. Fighting using groundwork or groundfighting exclusively.

open skill. Also called an open-ended skill or movement, a movement performed in an unpredictable pattern, in an uncontrolled environment, or in an environment with wide parameters. An example would be using a technique or movement when engaged in randori, which is an open-ended skill.

optimal. The most favorable degree or amount of something for obtaining a given result. For our purposes, when an athlete performs a technique with optimal skill, he is doing it in the most efficient manner that works best for him in the situation for which it is intended.

osaekomi waza. "Restrain, keep down, immobilize, pin, or control." Komi translates to "put into or to apply," and waza translates to "technique." This word is used in judo to denote a pinning technique. In Japanese jujutsu, the general application of an osae waza was to immobilize the opponent facedown on the ground or mat. With the advent of Kodokan judo in the early twentieth century, osae waza came to be used in contests for immobilizing the opponent on his back.

owaza. These are large or "big" throwing techniques that are large body movements such as uchi mata, tai otoshi, and seoi nage. These are different from kowaza and "minor" techniques such as foot sweeps and hooks using less large body movement.

pace. How fast or slow the attacker and defender move about the mat. This is also called tempo.

phase. A part of a connected series of movements.

plantar flexion. The action of the ankle joint when the foot moves downward and away from the leg (as in pointing the toes when performing a throwing technique).

position. Where an athlete's body is at any given time on the mat, and where he is relative to his opponent at any given time.

posting. Takes place when an athlete positions himself on the top of his head, places his hand on the mat, or extends his leg to place his foot on the mat in order to provide a stable base for himself in groundfighting. In essence, posting on top of the head, extending the arm and placing the hand on the mat, or extending the leg and placing the foot on the mat create a wider base area for increased stability. See **base**.

power. The measured rate of doing work. Force multiplied by the distance an object or body is moved.

power peak. The highest point in the trajectory of a throwing technique.

practice. The generic name used to describe the time allotted for a group of people to get together to train in an athletic activity, most often under the direction of a coach or senior member of the group. An effective practice will focus on the student or athlete learning, retaining, and mastering technical skill. A good practice will also provide the athletes with a physically challenging workout most suitable to the age, physical abilities, and health of the students or athletes. An effective practice must be appropriate to the skill level, maturity, and physical abilities of the students on the mat.

progression of skill. This is when learning takes place sequentially; one thing leads to another, and that thing leads to the next thing in a logical progression. The student progresses from the basic application of a skill on to more advanced applications of that skill. See **sequential teaching**.

proximity. How close the bodies of the attacker and defender are to each other. This is the space between the attacker and defender, often measured by how far the shoulders and hips are from each other.

randori. Randori is "free practice." While the name implies freedom of choice in movement, it is very much a drill. Randori must always be supervised and have a purpose. This is the same definition for a drill. Randori in judo is the same as a scrimmage in football or a sparring session for a boxer. It is training and not a contest, as in a tournament. Randori is an example of an open-ended drill.

rate of success. The frequency and regularity with which a skill is used with a successful outcome. If a specific technique often results in a score or ippon, that skill has a high ratio of success. This also relates to using the right movement or technique at the right time during a match. An athlete may have a specific technique or movement he uses in a specific situation with good results, and he knows he can count on it when he needs it. This move has a high rate of success. This is similar to a tokui waza, or favorite technique, but applied in a more tactical way. Conversely, an athlete will have other techniques that have a low rate of success and he won't use them. See **tokui waza**.

reaction time. The amount of time it takes for a body to respond to a stimulus. See **movement time**.

reflex. An action or movement performed as a response to a stimuli without conscious thought.

renraku waza. "Combination techniques." The attacker hits in with an initial throwing attack that may be a real attempt to throw his opponent or it may be a feint, but the opponent blocks or evades the attack. The attacker then switches to another throw, but in the opposite direction of the initial attack.

renzoku waza. "Continuation techniques." In this series of movements, the follow-up attack is a continuation of the initial attack. The attacker will either make a real initial attempt to throw his opponent or use a feint to elicit a response. As the defender evades or blocks the initial throwing attack, the attacker will hit in immediately with a second throw as a continuation of the initial attacking movement and often in the same direction as the initial attack.

repetition. Performing a movement more than once.

rides. The purpose of a ride is to control the opponent for as long as necessary in order to apply a submission technique or pin in groundfighting.

rotation. The act of one body or object turning around another body or object.

sankaku. A triangle: san translates to "three" and kaku translates to "corner" or "angle." As used in sankaku jime (triangle strangle) or sankaku gatame (triangle pin).

sensei. This term refers to a teacher. The word translates to "teacher" or "professor" and is also used to describe an elderly person, doctor, or scholar. Sensei refers to a person of high standing in the field of teaching or in the community. In the vernacular use of the term, it means "coach" but with the caveat that it is said with respect. This title is most often applied to experienced coaches, but it is commonly used to address any instructor. When visiting another judo club, it is considered good etiquette to address the head coach (as well as any black belt on the mat) as "sensei."

seoi. "Carry over the back" (se means "back," and oi means "to carry") and is used to describe the throwing techniques classified as seoi nage. It is commonly translated as "shoulder" when used in connection with the English translation of the names of these throws. Seoi nage describes the action of the movement in this throwing technique and means "carry over the back throw."

sequence. A connected group of movements usually with one part of the movement being dependent on the previous part of the movement.

sequential teaching. A technique used in teaching motor skills and movement but can be used in the teaching of any skill. A skill is taught in a sequence with each part of the movement building on the preceding part and necessary for the part that is next to come. The student progresses from one layer to the next until the student is able to achieve mastery of the basic structure of the skill. See **progression of skill**.

shiai. This term implies a trial of skill and means "coming together to test." Judo tournaments are referred to as shiai, implying that they are not fights without regard to rules but rather a trial of skill. See **shobu**.

shime waza. A term used to describe strangling techniques. Shime translates to "tighten, press, squeeze, or close." Waza translates to "technique." In the early period of judo's development, the neck, throat, and trunk of the body were the targets of shime waza. The idea was to squeeze a part of an opponent's body in order to restrict or shut off the supply of blood or air, or to restrict his breathing in any way. In the early part of the twentieth century, the contest rules of judo were changed so that the action of squeezing the body (dojime or "body squeezing") was no longer permitted and only the neck and throat remained as targets of shime waza. There are two ways to restrict an opponent's air intake: attack the carotid arteries, cutting off the blood supply (carrying oxygen) to the brain, or attack the trachea to obstruct or shut the airway. Restricting the flow of blood by squeezing or constricting the carotid arteries is a strangle according to the strict definition, and obstructing or blocking the airway is a choke. It is common to refer to shime waza as either a "choking technique" or a "strangle technique."

shintai. "Advance and retreat." Specifically, to advance and retreat in a linear pattern (either front and back or laterally). A generic translation is "footwork" as this term refers in a general sense to all footwork used in judo.

shisei. "Posture." The actual structure or how erect a person stands or how a human body presents itself is "posture." This term is also used in a general way to imply an athlete's stance.

shizentai. "Natural posture." Shizentai is an upright posture allowing the athletes the most freedom of movement and control of their own bodies. Shizen implies "natural" and tai refers to "the posture of the body."

shobu. "Win or lose" or "victory or defeat." The term implies victory in a contest and, often, a fight. See **shiai**.

shumatsu-undo. Cool-down exercises.

skill. The actual application of a technique. The optimal application of a technique or any movement. A movement pattern designed to meet the demands of a specific activity.

speed. The rate of a body's movement with no consideration of direction.

stability. The resistance of an object or body to being unbalanced, moved, or toppled.

stance. Foot placement and how an athlete stands combined with his posture. Stance is an integral part of posture and provides a base for an athlete when standing.

statics. The area of body mechanics concerning bodies at rest or moving at a constant velocity.

strength. The ability of a muscle to exert force against resistance.

style. The personal variation or adaptation of a technique or pattern of movement.

sukashi. The defensive action of avoiding an opponent's technique. Sukashi translates to "avoid."

tachi. This translates "to stand" and also implies how a person stands. Tachi-ai translates to "meet together for combat." So for general purposes these terms refer to "stance" as used in the martial arts. See **stance**.

taisabaki. A rotary, turning, or circling movement. "Tai" means "body" and "sabaki" implies "management" or "movement" and suggests preparation for getting into position for a subsequent movement.

takedown. A takedown's primary purpose is to take the opponent from a standing position to the mat and exert further control over him.

technique. The form or structure of something. How a specific movement is most commonly believed to be used or look like.

throw. To project an object or body in a specific direction through the air. This is what is meant when it is said that one athlete "throws" another athlete. The primary purpose of a throw is to put an opponent on the mat forcefully and with control. The hard and controlled landing from a throw can end a fight immediately, and this is why ippon is scored for a successfully executed throw.

timehold. Holding and controlling an opponent in osaekomi waza for a specified period of time is a "timehold." Gene LeBell was the first to use this term, as far as I know, back in the 1960s.

tokui waza. "Specialty technique." This is an athlete's go-to technique that has a high rate of success. See **rate of success**.

tori. The person applying a technique on his partner or opponent. This word translates to "taker" or "catcher" and implies the person catching his partner or opponent or taking part in the attacking action. See **uke**.

torque. Turning effect caused by a force around an axis.

trajectory. A body's flight path when it is thrown from a stable base standing.

transition. The action that takes place when the attacker takes his opponent from a standing position to the mat with a specific purpose in mind.

tsugi ashi. A shuffling or sliding footwork pattern, often at an angle (at the corners) or sideways (laterally) but sometimes in a straight line forward and backward. Tsugi means "successive" and implies a shuffling movement where one foot meets the other but the feet never cross. Ashi means "foot or leg" and implies the movement of the foot or a pattern.

tsukuri. This word implies "building," "constructing," or "forming" a technique. Tsukuri is often referred to as to "fit in" to the technique. The tsukuri action flows smoothly from kuzushi, and in reality there is an immediate and seamless transition from kuzushi to tsukuri when done correctly—so much so that it is hard to tell them apart if done optimally.

tsurite. The hand that lifts, traps, hooks, and generally manipulates the defender in a throwing technique. Tsuri translates to "lift or support" and te translates to "hand."

turnover. This word is used to describe rolling an opponent over onto his back, and this is an accurate description of what takes place. But a turnover is actually a breakdown in application, taking an opponent from a stable to an unstable position. See **breakdown**.

uchikomi. A drill done with a partner where an athlete repeatedly enters into the technique but does not finish it. When doing uchikomi for throwing techniques, the emphasis is on developing a fast rotational or turning movement of the hips and body as the attacker enters the technique. Uchi translates to "striking or hitting" and komi translates to "apply." See **butsukari**.

uke. The person a technique is applied to. This word translates to "receive" or "be the subject of something" and implies that this person is receiving the technique or having it applied to him. See **tori**.

ukemi. The primary method of safety used in judo is commonly called breakfalls. Ukemi implies "the body receiving the mat," with uke meaning "receiving" and mi meaning "body."

uki. "Straddle, float, or skim along the surface." This word is used in names of techniques such as uki otoshi (floating technique) or uki gatame (straddle pin). Though it sounds similar, uki should not be confused with uke.

velocity. The rate of a body's movement with controlled direction. The speed of a body in a specific direction. Velocity changes when the direction of movement changes.

waza. "Technique."

waza-ari. A score used in judo contests that denotes less than ippon. Waza translates to "technique" and ari translates to "almost." See **ippon**.

weight. The force of a body or object exerted by gravity.

REFERENCES

Bunasawa, Nori, and John Murray. *The Toughest Man Who Ever Lived*. Irvine, CA: Judo Journal and Innovations, 2007.

Carr, Gerry. *Mechanics of Sport*. Champaign, IL: Human Kinetics Publishing, 1997.

Cook, Gray. *Athletic Body in Balance*. Champaign, IL: Human Kinetics Publishing, 2005.

Daigo, Toshiro. *Kodokan Judo Throwing Techniques*. New York: Kodansha USA Publishing, 2016.

Draeger, Donn. *Modern Bujutsu & Budo*. New York: Weatherhill Publishers, 1997.

Gladwell, Malcom. *Outliers*. New York: Black Bay Books, 2013.

Gleeson, Geof. *All about Judo*. Cranford, UK: EP Publishing, 1984.

Gleeson, Geof. *Judo for the West*. Cranford, UK: A.S. Barnes and Company, 1967.

Gleeson, Geof. *Judo Inside Out*. Rutland, VT: Lepus Books, 1983.

Greene, Robert. *Mastery*. New York: Penguin Books, 2017.

Harrison, E.J. *Judo on the Ground*. London: W. Foulsham and Company, 1959.

Hepburn, James Curtis. *A Japanese and English Dictionary*. Tokyo: Charles E. Tuttle Publishing Company, 1987.

Hoare, Syd. *A History of Judo*. London: Yamagi Books, 2009.

Illustrated Kodokan Judo. Tokyo: Kodansha, 1964.

Inman, Roy. *The Judo Handbook*. New York: Rosen Publishing, 2008.

Inokuma, Isao, and Nobuyuki Sato. *Best Judo*. Tokyo: Kodansha International, 2009.

Ishikawa, Takahiko, and Donn Draeger. *Judo Training Methods*, Tokyo: Charles E. Tuttle Company, 1961.

Kano, Jigoro. *Kodokan Judo*. New York: Kodansha International, 2013.

Kawamura, Teizo, and Toshiro Daigo. *Kodokan New Japanese-English Dictionary of Judo*. Tokyo: Foundation of Kodokan Judo Institute, 2000.

Koizumi, Gunji. *My Study of Judo*. New York: Sterling Publishing, 1960.

Kotani, Sumiyuki, Yoshimi Osawa, and Yuichi Hirose. *Newaza of Judo*. Kobe: Koyano Bussan Kaisha, Ltd, 1973.

LeBell, Gene, and Laurie Coughran. *The Handbook of Judo*. New York: Cornerstone Library, 1975.

Leggett, Trevor, and Katsuhiro Watanabe. *Championship Judo*. London: W. Foulsham and Company, 1964.

McGinnis, Peter. *Biomechanics of Sport and Exercise*. Champaign, IL: Human Kinetics Publishing, 2013.

Moshanov, Andrew. *Judo from a Russian Perspective*. Vaihinigen an der Enz, Germany: Ipa-Verlag, 2004.

Musashi, Miyamoto. *A Book of Five Rings*. Translated by Victor Harris. New York: The Overlook Press, 1974.

Nater, Swen, and Ronald Gallimore. *You Haven't Taught Until They Have Learned*. Morgantown, WV: Fitness Information Technology Publishers, 2010.

Pulkkinen, Wayland. *The Sport Science of Elite Judo Athletes*. Guelph, Ontario: Pulkinetics, 2001.

Saylor, John, and Steve Scott. *Conditioning for Combat Sports*. Santa Fe, NM: Turtle Press, 2013.

Scott, Steve. *Coaching on the Mat*. Kansas City, MO: Welcome Mat Books, 2005.

Scott, Steve. *Drills for Grapplers*. Santa Fe, NM: Turtle Books, 2012.

Scott, Steve. *Winning on the Mat*. Santa Fe, NM: Turtle Press, 2011.

Sharkey, Brian. *Coaches' Guide to Sport Physiology*. Champaign, IL: Human Kinetics Publishing, 1986.

Stevens, John. *The Way of Judo*. Boston: Shambhala Publications, 2013.

Watanabe, Jiichi, and Lindy Avakian. *The Secrets of Judo*. Rutland, VT: Tuttle Publishing, 1960.

Wooden, John. *They Call Me Coach*. Chicago: Contemporary Books, 2004.

Yessis, Michael. *Build a Better Athlete*. Terre Haute, IN: Equilibrium Books, 2006.

Yessis. Michael. *Kinesiology of Exercise*. Indianapolis: Masters' Press, 1998.

ABOUT THE AUTHOR

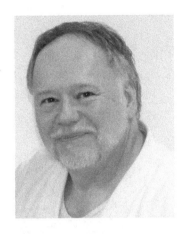

A graduate of the University of Missouri–Kansas City, Steve Scott holds high-dan grades in judo and Shingitai jujitsu and is a member of the US Sambo Hall of Fame. He has served as the US team coach at numerous international tournaments in judo, sambo, sport jujitsu, and submission grappling, including two IJF World Judo Championships (under 21), the IX Pan American Games for sambo, numerous PJU Pan American Judo Championships (for men, women, masters, and under 21), World Sambo Championships, and the International High School Judo Championships, as well as numerous international teams competing in Europe, North America, South America, and Asia. Steve served as the chairman of the Coach Development Program for the national governing body of judo, US Judo, Inc., and as the Junior (under 21) Development Program director / head coach for US Judo, Inc. Steve has conducted training camps at the US Olympic training centers as well as over 350 clinics and seminars across the United States. He founded the Welcome Mat Judo Club in 1969 and has developed hundreds of national and international medal winners as well as members of world, Pan American, and Olympic teams. Steve has served as the National Amateur Athletic Union Judo program chairman and is the innovator of the freestyle judo contest rules used by the AAU. Steve is married to Becky Scott, who is also active in judo and sambo and was the World and Pan American Games sambo champion.

BOOKS FROM YMAA

DVDS FROM YMAA

more products available from . . .

YMAA Publication Center, Inc. 楊氏東方文化出版中心

1-800-669-8892 • info@ymaa.com • www.ymaa.com

9 781594 396281